You Can Get
Pregnant
Over 40, Naturally II

*Overcoming infertility and recurrent miscarriage
in your late 30's and 40's naturally*

Sandy Robertson

Copyright © 2005, 2006, 2008, 2015 Sandy Robertson

All rights reserved. It is illegal to reproduce any portion of this material without authorization.

Printed in the United States of America

For information, contact:

SSE Online, LLC
P.O. Box 260744
Lakewood, CO 80226
www.getpregnantover40.com

Every effort has been made to make this information as complete and accurate as possible, but no warranty is implied. The material in this book is not intended to be a substitute for professional medical advice, diagnosis or treatment. Always seek the advice of a qualified health provider regarding your health or a medical condition.

Acknowledgements

I would like to thank all the women and couples who have openly shared with me their stories of infertility, pregnancy, miscarriage, childbirth, and finally, parenthood.

I would like to thank my husband who has been by my side every step of the way, and of course, I would like to thank my daughter for selecting me as her mother.

Contents

Acknowledgements iv

Introduction vii

Chapter 1 1
   Encouraging Information 1

Chapter 2 11
   Some Arguments Against Assisted Reproduction 11

Chapter 3 25
   My Specific Pregnancy Protocol 25

Chapter 4 101
   Fertility Bodywork 101

Chapter 5 107
   Alternative Techniques 107

Chapter 6 112
   Visualization, Meditation and Changing Your Pregnancy Mindset for Conception 112

Chapter 7 126
   Join a Support Group 126

Chapter 8 133
   All Stressed Up and Going Nowhere 133

Chapter 9 141
   How I Became My Own Therapist 141

Chapter 10 153

Putting it All Together *153*
A Typical Day On My Pregnancy Protocol *153*

Chapter 11 .... **158**
Just For Men *158*

Chapter 12 .... **171**
Preventing and Dealing with Miscarriage *171*

Chapter 13 .... **191**
"Do You Have Children??" How to Deal With All Those Tough Questions and Other Tough Situations *191*

Part II **201**

Chapter 14 .... **202**
How Did It Come To This? How My Past Experiences and Choices Led to Infertility *202*

Chapter 15 .... **207**
My Experience with Assisted Reproductive Technologies *207*

Chapter 16 .... **215**
My Experience with Recurrent Miscarriage *215*

Chapter 17 .... **221**
Success at Last! *221*

Chapter 18 .... **235**
The Joy of Being an Older Parent *235*

Afterword **239**

<u>Introduction</u>

This book is for those women who want to have a baby later in life without the use of assisted reproductive technologies. When I was trying to get pregnant over the age of 40, I ran into so much negativity, I thought it would be helpful to share my story with others who were also trying. I am living proof that it *can* be done. I got pregnant naturally at 43 and 11 months *with only one fallopian tube* and had a baby at 44.

I hope my story inspires you in an otherwise seemingly hopeless situation. Infertility is one of the most difficult challenges I have faced in my life. What I didn't know in the beginning of my journey that I do know now is I had more control over my fertility than I was led to believe by the medical professionals. I'm not saying there isn't a place for assisted reproductive technologies, but if you fall into the unexplained category and you're older in reproductive terms, my techniques can work for you. They are simple, and extremely good for your body, mind, and soul. In retrospect, my journey through infertility has actually improved my health and forced me to confront much of my past that acted as a roadblock to my success.

About the book format:

In the earlier editions of this book, I had my own story throughout each of the chapters. In this current edition, my story is now in "part two" at the end of the book. This was done primarily to consolidate the pregnancy protocols and research together.

Please note:

The material provided in this book is not intended to be a substitute for professional medical advice, diagnosis or treatment. Always seek the advice of a qualified healthcare provider regarding your health or medical condition. Everyone's situation and physical condition is different and I cannot guarantee that what worked for me will work for you. It is a good idea to seek the opinion of a reproductive endocrinologist if you've failed to conceive for over a year. Infertility can be caused by underlying conditions that require evaluation and treatment.

Chapter 1
Encouraging Information

Let's start with some encouraging information.

Before the days of birth control, it was quite common for women over 40 to have babies. If you talk to your grandparents or anyone who was of childbearing age before reliable family planning methods, it certainly wasn't unusual (and hardly newsworthy) for women to have a pregnancy over 40. It may have been their last child rather than their first, but obviously their bodies were capable.

I know you've heard it all before, the pregnancy statistics over 40 are "dismal". As far as I'm concerned, statistics are for statisticians. What about the fact that the number of unintended pregnancies in women between 40 and 44 is second only to teenagers? Many women in their 40's think they're too old to get pregnant, they get a little lax with their birth control, and bingo! I would venture to guess most women over 40 aren't trying to get pregnant (and many have had sterilization procedures). I wonder what would happen to those statistics if all women over 40 *tried* to get pregnant. I think we'd all be surprised

It seems that many women who are in their late 30's and 40's have heard so much about how they're going to have trouble conceiving that they run to the nearest fertility clinic before giving Mother Nature a real chance. There are so many things you can do to enhance your fertility naturally.

I wish I had done my research *before* I started fertility treatments. Deep down, I knew I could get pregnant, but unfortunately I didn't trust my inner voice. As a result, I put myself through the physical pain and rigors of fertility treatments only to find out I had it in me all along. Don't make the same mistake I did. Give your body what it needs to succeed - you may be surprised what you're capable of!

Need Success Stories?

At the end of this book (spoiler alert!) I talk about a surprise pregnancy I had at the age of 49 (unfortunately I miscarried, but it just goes to show you that anything can happen). I thought it might be helpful to give you some encouragement by sharing stories of women who conceived naturally at ages that are considered almost impossible by the medical community. The Telegraph UK online interviewed Professor Kypros Nicolaides, a maternal-fetal medicine specialist. He told the paper that his own grandmother had a child at 53, and he was quoted to say, "The risks of late motherhood are completely exaggerated. There's an increased risk of Down syndrome but the vast majority of women have normal babies at 40 and completely normal pregnancies."[1] I have many more stories on my infertility-fertility blog of women who conceive naturally over 40 and 50, but here are some of my favorites:

Case #1 Debbie Hughes, England

What makes this case remarkable, as reported by the Daily Mail in the UK, is that Debbie got pregnant by surprise at

---

[1] Casilda, G. (2009, March 20). Older mothers: Late bloomers Many women in their forties are realising their dreams of motherhood. Retrieved March 3, 2015, from http://www.telegraph.co.uk/women/womens-health/5016916/Older-mothers-late-bloomers.html

the age of 53, and she was on the pill at the time.[2] She also admits to a "once in a blue moon" love life! What are the odds of that? Her pregnancy had a fairytale ending too. She carried to term and had a healthy baby after a natural delivery. At the time of her pregnancy she also had two grandchildren from her grown kids. After delivering her baby, she said her motherly instinct kicked in right away and her age just was not a factor (except to the doctors who, when finding out her age, automatically assumed she had donor eggs!)

Case #2 Dawn Brooke, England

This case was also reported by the Daily Mail.[3] Dawn Brooke gave birth at the age of 59 and was said to have a natural conception without fertility treatments. She gave birth to a healthy baby boy who grew up to love math and Harry Potter.

Case #3 Ruth Kistler

Ruth Kistler of Portland, Oregon gave birth to a daughter in Los Angeles, California, on October 18, 1956, at the age of 57. This was obviously before the days of fertility treatments!

---

[2] Weathers, H. (2012, January 27). Daily Mail. Retrieved from http://www.dailymail.co.uk/femail/article-2092968/My-gorgeous-little-accident-Debbie-amazed-doctors--mention-grandchildren--getting-pregnant-naturally-53-Pill-Here-shares-joy--exhaustion.html

[3] Kelly, T., & Clerkin, B. (2007, August 20). Daily Mail. Retrieved from http://www.dailymail.co.uk/news/article-476452/The-British-woman-worlds-oldest-natural-mother-59.html

Case #4 Louise Spicer

This is an interesting and remarkable story reported by The Mirror in the UK.[4] Louise Spicer suffered from infertility for years and had problems with blockages in her fallopian tubes for which she underwent surgery. She tragically suffered an ectopic pregnancy and later underwent IVF which failed. Thinking she was going through menopause at the age of 42, she and her husband (18 years her senior) found out she was pregnant and after a successful pregnancy she delivered a healthy baby. At the age of 44, she got pregnant again by surprise and delivered a healthy baby boy. If that wasn't remarkable enough, she got pregnant with twins (again by surprise) at the age of 46 and delivered two healthy girls.

Case #5 Anthea Burns

This case was reported by The Courier Mail in Australia.[5] Anthea Burns conceived naturally and had a healthy baby boy at the age of 50. Her husband was 54. After being told a year earlier that she was in menopause, and her husband was told that he had "couch potato sperm" they spontaneously conceived their son.

Case #6 Susan Samulski

As reported by the Toronto Star, Susan Samulski and her husband underwent IVF and had three children when they thought their family was complete. Twelve years later, at the age of 47, thinking she was either going through menopause (or worse, worried that her symptoms were

---

[4] Mirror. (2012, July 2). Retrieved from http://www.mirror.co.uk/news/real-life-stories/louise-and-bernand-spicer-ivf-joy-1050813
[5] Weston, P. (2011, June 5). Courier Mail. Retrieved from http://www.couriermail.com.au/lifestyle/parenting/anthea-burns-is-a-mum-to-be-at-50-and-all-without-ivf/story-e6frer7o-1226069328270

caused by a terminal illness) she found out she had spontaneously conceived. She gave birth to a healthy boy who they named "Zenon" which means "gift from God". [6]

Case #7 Giovanni Ciardi

As reported by the Daily Mail, This Italian woman amazed doctors by getting pregnant at 54 and having a successful pregnancy and a healthy baby girl. She was still having periods and thought the cessation of her menses was due to menopause. When she started feeling nauseous she suspected she might be pregnant. [7]

Case #8 Arcelia Garcia

This 54 year old women and her 60 year old husband had triplets without the use of fertility drugs or fertility treatments. As reported by the LA Times, Ms. Garcia said, "to receive a child, no woman is too old". Ms. Garcia considered her triplets a big wonderful surprise. [8]

Case #9 Natural Pregnancy at 50 After Failed IVF

In Japan, a 50 year old woman previously underwent multiple IVF cycles between the ages of 46-48 with no success. She discontinued fertility treatments due to psychological stress, anxiety, depression, irritability, fatigue and grief. Three months after she turned 50, she returned to the same clinic and was 8 weeks pregnant

---

[6] Rushowy, K. (2009, February 21). Toronto Star. Retrieved from
http://www.thestar.com/life/parent/2009/02/21/baby_name_surprise_gift_from_god.html
[7] Pisa, N. (2010, April 15). Daily Mail. Retrieved from
http://www.dailymail.co.uk/news/article-1278059/Italian-woman-shocks-doctors-falling-pregnant-aged-54--NATURALLY.html
[8] LA Times. (2011, January 11). Retrieved from
http://articles.latimes.com/2000/jan/11/news/mn-53830

completely naturally. She carried to term and had a healthy baby. This published case study concluded: "Stopping infertility treatment might be a viable alternative for achieving pregnancy in similarly psychologically-challenged infertile women."[9] I whole heartedly agree with the conclusion of that study!

Now all of the cases cited above were women who conceived naturally in their late 40's and well into their 50's. If I were to write about women who conceived naturally just in their 40's, I would have to write a completely new book devoted to the subject!

Can you have a safe pregnancy over 40?

When I was trying to conceive over the age of 40, I was bombarded with all of the negative outcomes. Everything I read talked about how women over 40 suffer higher miscarriage rates, higher stillbirth rates and higher rates of birth defects. I went out of my way to avoid reading about the doom and gloom of pregnancy over 40. When I finally got pregnant with my daughter, the well-meaning medical professionals added insult to injury by scaring me half to death by constantly reminding me that I was considered to be "advanced maternal age" and I had endless ultrasounds and every prenatal test in the book. I was counseled with genetic testing, and told that after my delivery (which could likely be a C-Section), I might need a hysterectomy if they couldn't get the placenta out. As it turns out, I had a completely normal pregnancy and a completely normal delivery with no interventions at all. Best of all, my daughter was a full term healthy baby.

---

[9] Matsubayashi H, Iwasaki K, Hosaka T, Sugiyama Y, Suzuki T, Izumi S, Makino T., Spontaneous conception in a 50-year old woman after giving up in-vitro-fertilization (IVF) treatments: involvement of the psychological relief in successful pregnancy. Tokai J Exp Clin Med. 2003 Apr;28(1):9-15.

Let's look at the facts about birth defects and other pregnancy complications:

What is the rate of Down Syndrome?

Most of the babies with Down Syndrome are born to women under the age of 35. If you are 40 years old, your chance of having a baby with Down Syndrome is only 1% and if you are 45 your chances are only 3.3%. So, yes, the risk increases, but it's not as high as you might be led to believe. The vast majority of babies are born normal.[10]

Do Women Over 40 Have More Pregnancy Complications or Worse Fetal Outcomes?

One of the biggest risk factors for pregnancy complications seems to be your weight rather than your age. According to the Life Issues Institute:

"In women of normal weight over 40, there was no difference in high blood pressure, no increase in large babies, no increase in fetal death rate, no more distress at delivery. Women of normal weight over 40 did have a little more diabetes and had a few more Caesarean sections. But their infant outcome was no different from that of the younger women."[11]

Additionally, the American Journal of Perinatology reported that even women over the age of 50 who became pregnant with donor eggs didn't have a significantly higher

---

[10] Down Syndrome Risk Factors. (2014, April 19). Retrieved March 3, 2015, from http://www.mayoclinic.org/diseases-conditions/down-syndrome/basics/risk-factors/CON-20020948

[11] Life Issues Institute (1996, July 18). [Radio broadcast]. Cincinnati: (citing journal Obstetrics and Gynecology "Pregnancy After Forty Years of Age" by Dr. Spellacy and colleagues)

rate of complications than women under the age of 42 and actually do pretty well. The study found women over age 50 had similar rates of complications, such as gestational diabetes and preterm labor, as women under age 42 who became pregnant after receiving donated eggs. And although the older women had slightly higher rates of high blood pressure, that difference was small, and may have been due to chance.[12]

Did You Know Some Birth Defects Are LESS Common in Women Over 40?

The Society for Maternal-Fetal Medicine reported that major congenital malformations were 40% less likely in pregnant women over the age of 35. There were lower rates of brain, kidney and abdominal wall defects.[13]

Childhood Outcomes Better In Older Mothers

As reported in The Journal of Family Healthcare (UK): "The Royal College of Pediatrics and Child Health conference has suggested that children born to mothers over 40 are healthier and brighter than those of younger women. The offspring of older women are less likely to have accidents or need hospital care and more likely to have been vaccinated early. They will also develop a broader vocabulary from a young age and achieve higher scores in IQ tests in a range of measures up to the age of five." The head of the study, Dr. Alastair Sutcliffe said negative publicity surrounding the rise of older mothers was based on the physical risks of pregnancy and childbirth

---

[12] Daniel H. Kort, MD (CUMC); Jennifer Gosselin, PhD (CUMC); Janet M. Choi, MD (CUMC); Melvin H. Thornton, MD; Jane Cleary-Goldman, MD (Mount Sinai Medical Center); and Mark V. Sauer, MD (CUMC).February 2012 issue of the American Journal of Perinatology.

[13] Goetzinger KR, et al "Advanced maternal age and the risk of major congenital anomalies: survival of the fittest?" SMFM 2014; Abstract 34.

Encouraging Information

but argued that: "We have clear evidence that there are more desirable outcomes for children of older mothers compared with younger ages. We can reassure these older women that their children are probably better off. The big question is why. Older mothers appear to have good parenting skills, they may be less impulsive, calmer and have more life experience that better equips them for the role. More women are giving birth at older ages, this isn't going to go away, they are deferring motherhood for many reasons."[14]

So the takeaway here is:

Yes, there are increases in Down Syndrome and some pregnancy complications in pregnant women over 40, however they are not huge increases. My pregnancy protocol later in this book will help prepare your body for a healthy pregnancy.

---

[14] Older Mums Less Accident Prone Claim Health Researchers. (2012). The Journal Of Family Healthcare UK ,(2012, May 22). Retrieved March 3, 2015, from www.jfhc.co.uk

Chapter 2
Some Arguments Against Assisted Reproduction

Obviously, I'm an advocate of conceiving naturally especially since I went through years of fertility treatments only to have my best success following an all-natural protocol. There are many reasons to think twice before jumping into fertility treatments:

Higher Incidence of Abnormalities

In all fairness, I should start by saying that the vast majority of babies conceived through assisted reproductive techniques are normal. However, there may be a higher incidence of certain birth defects and cognitive delays in babies conceived through IVF. One study found:
"IVF independently contributes a significant risk of congenital malformation in addition to known maternal factors. In particular, defects of the eye, heart and genitourinary system are more likely in infants born after IVF. "[15] Another study found: "Compared with spontaneous conception, IVF treatment overall was not associated with autistic disorder but was associated with a small but statistically significant increased risk of mental retardation"[16]

---

[15] Lorraine I. Kelley-Quon, M.D., M.S.H.S., Chi-Hong Tseng, Ph.D., Carla Janzen, M.D., Ph.D. and Stephen B. Shew, M.D., Congenital Malformations Associated with Assisted Reproductive Technology: A California Statewide Analysis. (2012, October 20). Retrieved March 16, 2015, from:
https://aap.confex.com/aap/2012/webprogram/Paper17831.html
[16] Sandin S, Nygren KG, Iliadou A, Hultman CM, Reichenberg A., Autism and mental retardation among offspring born after in vitro fertilization., JAMA. 2013 Jul 3;310(1):75-84. doi: 10.1001/jama.2013.7222.

Most experts agree that more study needs to be done to find out if some abnormalities are due to the procedures themselves or if it might have something to do with the fact that people undergoing IVF probably have other anatomical/medical issues that could contribute to the findings.

Placenta Previa

Placenta Previa has been found to be more common in IVF pregnancies[17]. It is a condition where the embryo attaches too low on the uterine wall and can either partially or fully cover the cervix leading to a number of complications. One explanation why this complication might be more common with IVF is that implantation rates may be higher when the embryo is placed lower down in the uterus.

Success Rates – Not What They Seem?

One of the first questions potential fertility patients have is: What are the IVF success rates? It is going to vary widely between different fertility clinics. However, you should be aware that there are a number of things that can influence success rates such as a few discussed below:

1. Selection criteria - Some IVF clinics have strict criteria related to age, pre-existing conditions, etc. and only the patients with the highest likelihood of success are accepted into their IVF program. This can boost their success rates substantially. Some clinics have even been known to refer tougher cases to clinics with lower

---

[17] Romundstad LB, Romundstad PR, Sunde A, von Düring V, Skjaerven R, Vatten LJ.Increased risk of placenta previa in pregnancies following IVF/ICSI; a comparison of ART and non-ART pregnancies in the same mother,Hum Reprod. 2006 Sep;21(9):2353-8. Epub 2006 May 25.

selection criteria. Dr. Mark Sauer said in his interview with *Frontine*: "Success rates are difficult, because everyone looks at a success rate as the baby for which they are trying so hard to achieve. They don't usually question the number. They don't ask what that really means to a program. For instance, if you lie two programs side by side and you see discrepancy between the programs' success rates, the automatic assumption is that one program is better than the other, and that's really not true in most cases. Programs are always different. They may treat different types of patients. If a program wants to maintain a very high success rate, they can and do literally select the best patients to treat. On the same hand, the competitors who may not get those best patients, a new program, for instance, in a marketplace, may be sort of stuck treating patients that other groups won't treat, which will automatically lower their success rates. So it's Catch-22. You can't really get out from under that unless you start selecting out only the best patients…each program director is faced with a very daunting task of trying to make a decision as to who they are going to treat, with the full knowledge, it's no secret, that the harder the cases, the lower the chance of success, and the more it may overall hurt the image of the program ..."[18]

2. Implanting a large number of embryos - we all know about the well-publicized cases of women having six and seven babies, however even a twin pregnancy has the potential to be more complicated than a singleton. Transferring a large number of embryos certainly will result in a higher success rate, but at what cost?

3. Cancellation of "poor response" cycles - Some clinics may cancel a cycle when only a few follicles develop as this may lower the probability of success.

---

[18] Interview, Dr. Mark Sauer. In Frontline.PBS.

4. Waiting lists - Some clinics may have waiting lists where the patients with the best probability of success are moved to the top.

Procedural Risks

Like all procedures, assisted reproduction has its own risks such as allergies to medications, hormonal swings from fertility drugs, infection around the drug injection sites, injury to abdominal structures (i.e. bowel, bladder, etc.) at the time of egg retrieval, pain, and bruising.

More Tubal Pregnancies with IVF

There is an increased risk of having a tubal pregnancy after IVF[19] (something I know all too well since I had two of them). It's difficult to know for sure why there is a higher incidence of tubal pregnancies with this procedure. It may be as a result of the type of catheter used during the embryo transfer, it may be a result of the embryo moving up into the tube from the uterus after the transfer, or it may be because the woman has some tubal scarring or other abnormality that might make the it difficult for the embryo to come back down into the uterus to implant.

Lab Mix-Ups

I had an interesting incident when we first started going through fertility treatments and we were trying inseminations. I went in for my insemination after my husband gave his "donation". After signing in at the doctor's office, I waited and waited. The receptionist kept giving me these weird looks and after I waited an hour and

---

[19] Malak M, Tawfeeq T, Holzer H, Tulandi T.
Risk factors for ectopic pregnancy after in vitro fertilization treatment.
J Obstet Gynaecol Can. 2011 Jun;33(6):617-9.

a half, the doctor himself called me into his office. He sheepishly told me there was a "mix up" in the lab and they had to cancel my insemination. The nurse jokingly says, "We wouldn't want a baby that doesn't look anything like you, now would we?" I sat there somewhat stunned, thinking, *"EXCUSE ME?? You mean to tell me my husband's sperm is floating around in the wrong pipette? And even worse, some other guy's sperm was in my pipette?!"* Well, in their defense, at least the lab technician admitted to the error. I really could have had someone else's baby. I still wonder if my husband's sperm might have been given to another woman. In retrospect, it really does make me think about all of the things that can happen when you fool with Mother Nature. I know that some couples have no choice but to undergo fertility treatments, but it is a little worrisome that you really never know what's going on in the lab. Everything is microscopic, if something gets mislabeled.....it's all over (or you could have a major dilemma the rest of your life). The same holds true for couples undergoing IVF or donor cycles. You're placing all your trust in lab technicians who may or may not be following standard protocol when handling your specimens. There have been a number of cases reported in the media of women who were impregnated with the wrong sperm or wrong embryo.

The "Extra Embryo" Dilemma

When undergoing IVF, many couples have extra embryos which are frozen. Some actually have quite a few. You have a number of options. You could have them destroyed (basically, they thaw them out, then discard them). You could implant them to see if they "take". If you've completed your family, you could donate them. All of these things are hard decisions to make. I know one couple who did an IVF cycle with donor eggs from a 21 year old woman. They harvested quite a few eggs and they ultimately got pregnant with twins. There were four extra embryos left over that were frozen. There were quite a few complications during the twin pregnancy but fortunately, the twins were born healthy. The mother was advised not to get pregnant again because of some damage to her uterus. The couple had a major dilemma on their hands because they had four extra embryos and they could not undergo another procedure. They absolutely did not want to have the embryos discarded. The couple was saving up their money to implant the 4 frozen embryos but this time they were looking at using a surrogate. They may even need to do two cycles with a surrogate depending on whether or not their RE was willing to implant all four embryos at once or only a couple at a time. You can see how complicated this situation has become. In addition, if you donate your embryos to another couple and a pregnancy results, you will have to decide and agree upon whether or not you will stay anonymous, whether the child may contact you, etc.

If you can't make up your mind about what to do with your frozen embryos, you can continue to have them stored, however this can be quite expensive and can amount to hundreds of dollars in ongoing storage fees.

The Safety Of Fertility Drugs

You may have heard about a possible link between fertility drugs and ovarian cancer. Some recent studies have shown no link between fertility drugs and ovarian cancer (the higher incidence of cancer among women who took fertility drugs was attributed to their underlying cause of infertility, not the drugs themselves). The basic theory of why fertility drugs may increase a women's risk for cancer is that the more ovulations a woman has in her lifetime, the higher the risk for cancer. Things that decrease the number of ovulations a woman has over a lifetime can decrease the risk for cancer. For example, if a woman is on birth control pills, if a woman becomes pregnant, or if a woman breastfeeds, ovulation is suppressed and this lowers her risk. Even though ovarian cancer and fertility drugs cannot be linked, it should be mentioned that clomiphene (Clomid) has been associated with an increased risk of thyroid cancer[20].

Fertility drugs may also be bad for your oral health. The hormones in fertility drugs can cause gum inflammation and bleeding because of hormone receptors in these areas. "Women undergoing fertility treatments or IVF can be at a greater risk for gingivitis or gum disease. Research has found that women who used ovulation-inducing medications for more than three menstrual cycles had higher levels of gum inflammation and bleeding than women not on the drugs."[21]

Some fertility drugs may actually *decrease* fertility. Clomid can cause vaginal dryness and cause changes in the quality and quantity of cervical mucus[22]. Even when this drug was used with inseminations (to by-pass hostile mucus), pregnancy rates weren't significantly better than those who tried naturally. Other frequently prescribed drugs have also been found to be of little or no benefit. For example, gluticosteriods which have an anti-inflammatory

---

[20] C.G. Hannibal, A. Jensen, H. Sharif and S.K. Kjaer, Risk of thyroid cancer after exposure to fertility drugs: results from a large Danish cohort study, Hum. Reprod. (2008) 23 (2): 451-456. doi: 10.1093/humrep/dem381 First published online: December 6, 2007

[21] Marsh, D. (n.d.). During Your Pregnancy: Dental Health Care. Retrieved April 1, 2015, from http://www.todaysdentistry.com.au/did-you-know/during-your-pregnancy-taking-care-of-your-dental-health/

22 Marchini M, Dorta M, Bombelli F, Ruspa M, Campana A, Dolcetta G, Radici E., Effects of clomiphene citrate on cervical mucus: analysis of some influencing factors. Int J Fertil. 1989 Mar-Apr;34(2):154-9.

effect have been used to enhance uterine receptivity to an embryo. These drugs have not been found to be effective and, if the woman should become pregnant, little is known how they might negatively affect the pregnancy.[23]

Finally, a recent study made a connection between fertility drugs and childhood cancer. The risk of developing the rare acute myeloid leukemia was increased 2.3-fold by the drugs. The most common type, acute lymphoblastic leukemia, showed a two-to six-fold increase.[24]

It scares me to think about all the drugs and hormones I was pumping into my system while undergoing fertility treatments. Aside from the previously mention risks, fertility drugs can lead to hyperstimulation of the ovaries (which I experienced twice when going through IVF). Although I had a mild form of the condition, it can be quite severe and may require hospitalization.

If you should decide to use fertility drugs, ask your doctor specifically about the risks. New research is being done all the time and just because we don't know about possible risks now, it doesn't necessarily mean these drugs are safe.

The good news is that if you do become pregnant, new information is emerging that shows pregnancy over the age of 40 may actually reduce the risk of endometrial cancer (cancer of the uterus).[25] Endometrial cancer rates may be reduced because the "bad" cells may shed along with the

---

[23] Center for the Advancement of Health. (2007, March 6). Steroid Use Fails To Boost Pregnancy Rates In Infertility Treatments. ScienceDaily. Retrieved March 30, 2015 from www.sciencedaily.com/releases/2007/03/070302082350.htm
[24] Fertility drugs more than double childhood cancer risk, scientists say. (2013, April 24). Retrieved March 30, 2015, from http://www.foxnews.com/health/2012/04/24/fertility-drugs-more-than-double-childhood-cancer-risk-scientists-say
[25] Veronica Wendy Setiawan et al, Age at Last Birth in Relation to Risk of Endometrial Cancer, Am. J. Epidemiol. (2012) doi: 10.1093/aje/kws129 First published online: July 23, 2012

placenta and other uterine contents at the time of delivery. Ovarian cancer risk may also be lower in women having their first pregnancy over 40.[26]

Cost

When all was said and done, my husband and I spent approximately $25,000 on fertility treatments only to walk away with nothing (not to mention one less fallopian tube). The average IVF cycle costs well over $10,000 (maybe more or less depending on where you live and which clinic you go to). If you have insurance that pays for assisted reproduction, consider yourself lucky because many people do not. In retrospect, I think about how that $25,000 we spent on failed fertility treatments could have been a college fund for my daughter, and it's amazing how financially conservative we are with every other aspect of our life. I can't think of any other medical procedure done on basically healthy people that is so risky, expensive, and success is far from guaranteed. It's just that you want a baby so bad, you're willing to do *anything* and that desperation can lead to hasty and sometimes impulsive decision making. Most of us have been so conditioned to seek medical and pharmaceutical help for every disorder, we don't even consider the natural route. It certainly makes sense to try the free, natural and healthy methods before giving away your hard-earned money and exposing yourself to a multitude of complications.

---

[26] Penmann, D. (2002, March 25). Later motherhood "reduces ovarian cancer risk" Retrieved April 1, 2015, from http://www.newscientist.com/article/dn2082#.VRxSZuHEvIU

The Increasing Number of Women Conceiving Naturally After IVF

It has been recently reported that there is an increasing rate of women who have had one child through IVF who spontaneously conceive their second child naturally. This could be for a number of reasons. First, it is possible that these women would have conceived their first child naturally if they would have given it more time. Second, IVF may be recommended for unexplained infertility more often now than in the past. Third, let's not forget the obvious. Women who have finally succeeded in having their baby don't have the stress of facing infertility, and the rigors of IVF. I'm sure there are many couples out there who examine their choice to pursue assisted reproduction only to find out they had the ability to get pregnant and carry to term on their own. In Australia, it was reported that 1/3 of couples who have a baby through IVF conceive a subsequent pregnancy naturally.[27]

Does High FSH Mean You Have to Have IVF with Donor Eggs?

FSH stands for follicle stimulating hormone and it rises as your body tries harder to develop eggs which may indicate the start of ovarian failure. Many women over the age of 40 have been told that their FSH levels are on the high side. Usually, fertility doctors want the FSH to be under 10. However, there are recorded cases of women getting pregnant with their own eggs with FSH levels that were even over 100! For example, The Oxford Journals Human Reproduction reported on three cases of women who had

---

[27] Wynter, K., McMahon, C., Hammarberg, K., McBain, J., Boivin, J., Gibson, F. and Fisher, J. (2013), Spontaneous conceptions within two years of having a first infant with assisted conception. Australian and New Zealand Journal of Obstetrics and Gynaecology, 53: 471–476. doi: 10.1111/ajo.12112

successful pregnancies with their own eggs with FSH levels that would be considered "off the chart" and most doctors would have only given them the option of donor eggs. In one case, a 46 year old got pregnant with an FSH of 22. The other cases in the report were a 36 year old with an FSH of 143 and a 35 year old with an FSH of 105. The study reported: "there does not appear to be a ceiling on the FSH concentration where conception in a woman with incipient ovarian failure is not possible. Furthermore, they can be advised that there is at least one precedent for temporary reversal of apparent overt menopause with successful delivery in women up to the age of 45 years".[28]

Stress

Later, I talk about how stress can contribute to infertility and even miscarriage. However, infertility treatments themselves are an extremely stressful experience. While undergoing treatments, your entire life completely revolves around when you have to take your medications, when you ovulate, and when you go in for procedures. What I found particularly stressful is that the actual date when you go in (whether it's inseminations or IVF) depends upon when your follicles develop. You have to be ready at the drop of a hat to run into the RE's office for a procedure. If you're trying to hold down a job, it can be quite tricky to get time off work (especially if you want to keep your information confidential). I was working at the beginning of our fertility treatments (while we were undergoing inseminations), and I was constantly coming up with excuses about why I had to leave or take a day off work. When we started going through IVF, thankfully, I had quit

---

[28] Three pregnancies despite elevated serum FSH and advanced age, Oxford Journals Human Reproduction (2000) 15 (8): 1709-1712. doi: 10.1093/humrep/15.8.1709

my job. I don't know how I could have fit the rigors of IVF into my work schedule.

Going through IVF, whether you're working or not, has its own set of stressors. My husband had to give me the injections so he had to learn the process and had to be ready at specified intervals. Prior to the egg retrieval and the embryo transfer procedures, I was usually awake all night worrying about how the procedure would go. I would worry that the car was going to break down on the way to the fertility clinic or I would worry that there was going to be a snowstorm and somehow we couldn't get there. Even if I got to the clinic, I would worry if they'd be able to get my eggs out. Was it going to hurt? Were there going to be complications? Were there going to be enough fertilized embryos to do the transfer? You have so much invested in this one procedure (not just time, but of thousands of dollars) it's bound to be stressful in some way. Then there's the two week wait after the embryo transfer. It is absolutely agonizing. You overanalyze anything and everything. Did I feel a cramp? Does the spotting mean I'm pregnant and miscarrying? Why are my breasts sore or why aren't they sore? Is my baby going to be ok? And the list goes on. The medications that you're given during fertility treatments also put you on an emotional roller coaster ride. I frequently would feel rage or sadness for no reason at all. I commend my husband for putting up with my out-of-control emotions during that time.

For couples undergoing fertility treatments, the number one reason for dropping out is financial and the number two reason is stress.[29] One study found: "An unexpectedly high

---

[29] Kulkarni, G., Mohanty, N. C., Mohanty, I. R., Jadhav, P., & Boricha, B. G. (2014). Survey of reasons for discontinuation from in vitro fertilization treatment among couples attending infertility clinic. Journal of Human Reproductive Sciences, 7(4), 249–254. doi:10.4103/0974-1208.147491

percentage of couples who performed IVF discontinued the treatment before the three cycles that were offered. A majority of these discontinuations were due to psychological stress."[30]

Even if your procedure is successful, many IVF patients have to continue with progesterone shots or other medications. I had hyperstimulation of my ovaries and it was recommended that I take antihistamines to help reduce the fluid that accumulates with this condition. These antihistamines had to be taken three times per day, so I was in a constant state of drowsiness to the point that I was afraid to drive. I was also worried about whether or not these medications were going to hurt the baby (this was when I got pregnant through IVF before I miscarried). I had the additional trauma of having numerous pregnancy losses (and undergoing surgery for an ectopic). It's no wonder I couldn't take it anymore. Going through IVF was one of the worst experiences in my life. If only I had known then what I know now.

What about babies born through IVF, do we know what the psychological effects are?

According to Karen Melton, DH Psych, Prenatal & Birth Therapist (who counsels children born through IVF),

"In IVF we have a whole cast of characters involved in the pre-conception and conception phases who would not normally be there. We know in Prenatal & Peri-natal Psychology & Health (PPN) that even at the conception stage we are being influenced by the energetic field around us, and what is going on within it. That field is primarily

---

[30] Catharina Olivius, Barbro Friden, Gunilla Borg, Christina Bergh
Psychological aspects of discontinuation of in vitro fertilization treatment
Fertility and Sterility, Volume 81, Issue 2, February 2004, Pages 276

our mom and our parent's relationship/connection. Your child is having her own experience as she is navigating through this elaborate process. We need to gather much more information from children about how this is affecting them."

"An IVF conception is totally unique in that it is the only time a child is conceived with both the parents not present. There is a lot going on at conception, as we are:
- Coming into the physical body of our mother
- Beginning to grow our own body
- Entering into the field of our parents for the first time
- Coming into the ancestral lines of our parents, and into what our soul level commitment is with this family line in particular."

"Conception is a sacred event. The sacred is rarely included or acknowledged during medical procedures. We now have considerable understanding of the emotional/psychological aspects of early imprinting and this also needs to be included in the IVF process. It makes a lot of sense to me that IVF children would acutely feel the absence of their parent's presence at their conception. It is not possible for me at this stage to say what the effects of this kind of conception would have on these children in relation to their sense of relationship, sexuality, and spirituality. It may be that they are spiritually/energetically with their parents at conception even though the event itself is physically happening somewhere else. It will be fascinating to see this story unfold from the mouths of our babies and children."[31]

---

[31] Melton, K. (2012, July 12). How In-Vitro Fertilization (IVF) Can Affect Your Child. Retrieved March 3, 2015, from http://healyourearlyimprints.com/blog/?p=175

Chapter 3
My Specific Pregnancy Protocol

I spent years researching natural methods to enhance fertility. I read food and nutrition publications, medical studies, and I educated myself on natural treatments that would normalize hormonal levels, promote ovulation, and increase pelvic circulation. I continued to refine my diet and treatment regime until I came up with the winning formula.

One thing I kept running across in my research was something called "estrogen dominance". Estrogen dominance is when you have excess estrogen especially compared to progesterone. This can cause a number of fertility problems, including uterine fibroids and even endometriosis (and wouldn't you know it, suffered from both). I also learned there are environmental toxins called xenoestrogens. This literally means "foreign estrogen". These xenoestrogens mimic estrogen in your system contributing to estrogen dominance. Xenoestrogens are stored in the body for an extended period of time leading to a number of conditions which ultimately contribute to infertility. I have a list of xenoestrogens to avoid at the end of this chapter (under the "Things to Avoid" heading.)

Phytoestrogens, on the other hand, are plant based substances which also mimic estrogens (phytoestrogen means "plant estrogen"), however they are weaker and they differ from xenoestrogens because they are actually beneficial. Phytoestrogens bind with estrogen receptors keeping out the stronger more harmful estrogens (like xenoestrogens). Phytoestrogens are not stored in the body and are easily broken down. Later, in my "Fertility Diet" section, I give you a list of vegetables that are high in phytoestrogens.

Additionally, my research uncovered a group of hormone-like substances called prostaglandins which play a critical role in menstruation, conception, and pregnancy. There are different types of prostaglandins, some are helpful and some are harmful. Some prostaglandins assist the uterus and the fallopian tubes to contract which moves the egg to the portion of the tube where fertilization is most likely to occur. Prostaglandins also surge at the end of a menstrual cycle causing the corpus luteum of the ovary to shrink down which tells the body to start a new cycle.

You can see that there is a synchronistic orchestration of events that should occur in a normal cycle. If there is an overproduction of prostaglandins (with endometriosis, for example) and woman becomes pregnant or is pregnant, this could cause the uterine lining to shed ending in a miscarriage. Additionally, overproduction of prostaglandins could cause contractions so powerful that the egg moves too fast before conception can occur.

In terms of getting pregnant and staying pregnant, it is important to help your body manufacture and shift the balance to good prostaglandins by eating foods that create the building blocks for these substances. Specifically, you need to be consuming essential fatty acids since your body can't manufacture these by itself. Omega-3 fatty acids are particularly helpful. The three main forms are eicosapentaenoic acid (EPA), docosahexaenoic acid (DHA), and alpha-linolenic acid (ALA). EPA and DHA are considered long-chain forms of omega-3 and are found in fish, fish oil supplements, and algae extract. ALA, the short-chain form, is found in plant sources like walnuts, flax seed, canola and soybean oil, and, to a lesser degree, green leafy vegetables.

Not only will omega 3's help your body with hormone production, but if you do become pregnant, research has confirmed that adding EPA and DHA to the diet of pregnant women has a positive effect on visual and cognitive development of the baby. Studies have also shown that higher consumption of omega-3s may reduce the risk of allergies in infants. Omega-3 fatty acids have positive effects on the pregnancy itself. Increased intake of EPA and DHA has been shown to help prevent pre-term labor and delivery, lower the risk of preeclampsia and may increase birth weight. Omega-3 deficiency increases the mother's risk for depression.[32]

My Fertility Diet section includes foods that are high in Omega-3's and this is one area where you should consider taking a supplement (see more in supplements later in this chapter).

What about high FSH?

I previously quoted a study which reported on women who conceived with their own eggs with an FSH over 100. After I discontinued fertility treatments, I never had my FSH checked because I didn't want more discouraging information clouding my mindset. I knew I was going to get pregnant even if the odds were against me. So, what can you do to lower FSH naturally? Here are my top 3 recommendations which are further addressed in my pregnancy protocol parts I-III:

---

[32] Omega-3 Fish Oil and Pregnancy. (2014, December 1). Retrieved March 12, 2015, from http://americanpregnancy.org/pregnancy-health/omega-3-fish-oil/

1. Increase pelvic circulation: hormones and oxygen travel through the circulatory system. You can visit a qualified massage therapist for a pelvic massage, or this is something you can perform on yourself (see my chapter on Fertility Bodywork and I have a video through my website getpregnantover40.com.)
2. Increase the good fats in your diet. Essential fatty acids help your body manufacture hormones (my fertility diet has many sources).
3. Get sufficient protein. Hormones are made of proteins. There are plenty of sources of vegetable protein as discussed in the next section.

My Pregnancy Protocol -Part I
My Fertility Diet

My diet consisted of 8-12 servings of hormone regulating fruits and vegetables and a number of seeds, nuts, beans and proteins (mostly vegetable protein, but some meat, fish and poultry as well). This may require a major shift in your eating. I really had to plan ahead and start eating the vegetables in the morning to get all my servings in. I tried to vary what types of vegetables I ate. Every Sunday, I would go to the grocery store and buy all of my produce to eat throughout the week. I know that many experts on food and nutrition strongly recommend organic fruits and vegetables (these are grown without pesticides which can be xenoestrogens). Sometimes I bought organic, however many times I did not. I think for most people, just eating more fruits and vegetables would be a major improvement in their diet whether or not they're organic. According to The Environmental Working Group, the following produce has been found to be the most contaminated with pesticides, so if you are going to buy organic, these should be at the top of your list: apples, peaches, nectarines, strawberries, grapes, celery, spinach, sweet bell peppers, cucumbers, cherry tomatoes, snap peas, potatoes, hot peppers, kale, and collard greens. [33] Be sure to wash all your fruits and vegetables thoroughly to remove any unhealthy residue (I would use a solution of white vinegar and water to wash all produce).

A note about convenience – If I had to cook every day, I probably wouldn't have stuck to this diet. I would designate Sunday as my cooking day and make a big platter of vegetables I would store in the refrigerator. I would eat a portion of each daily. You can vary the vegetables you

---

[33] EWG's 2015 Shopper's Guide to Pesticides in Produce. (2015, January 1). Retrieved April 10, 2015, from http://www.ewg.org/foodnews/summary.php

eat and you can add some that are not listed below. The main thing here is to have at *least* 8 servings and if possible 10-12.

Here is a summary of my diet:

Flax Seeds

Flax seeds are a great hormone regulator and help with estrogen metabolism.[34] I would grind them up in my coffee grinder and store them in the freezer (you can also buy them already ground – ask your grocer for "flax meal"). You should keep flax seeds either refrigerated or frozen because their natural oils can easily spoil. I would take about 2 tablespoons of flax seeds every day. Flax seeds contain something called lignans. Lignans are phytoestrogens (mentioned above) which, again, bind to estrogen receptors blocking the effects of the stronger more harmful estrogens. Flax seeds are also a great source of Omega-3 fatty acids which help your body manufacture the "good" prostaglandins.

Nuts

Nuts also contain many of the good fats that are excellent for your overall health and fertility. Almost all types of nuts are great, but eat in moderation since they're high in calories. I would usually have about a handful per day. Almonds and walnuts are particularly helpful and there may be additional benefits from eating walnuts for women with polycystic ovarian syndrome - PCOS. When you buy nuts, buy them raw (i.e. unroasted) and unsalted. The roasting process can spoil the beneficial oils. Also, be sure to keep them in the refrigerator to ensure the oils stay fresh

---

[34] Morris, D,PhD. (2007). Flax - A Health and Nutrition Primer. Retrieved March 6, 2015, from http://www.flaxcouncil.ca/english/pdf/FlxPrmr_4ed_Chpt4.pdf

(actually, they should be in the refrigerated section of the store – if they're not, don't buy them). I would also buy peanut butter, almond butter, hazelnut butter, and cashew butter for sandwiches (if you can't eat at home, this is a great lunch to pack). Be careful with some of the pre-packaged peanut butters because they contain partially hydrogenated vegetable oil to keep the oil from separating from the peanuts. You need to be sure you are buying the peanut butter that does not contain these harmful trans-fats. You will probably need to stir thoroughly when you buy the non-hydrogenated brands. Health food stores usually do not sell products with hydrogenated oils, so if you shop there, you can be fairly certain you're buying the healthiest version of the product.

Cruciferous Vegetables

Cruciferous vegetables include most listed below (i.e. broccoli, cauliflower, brussel sprouts and many of the greens.) Cruciferous vegetables have natural phytochemicals. The most active is something called DIM which is responsible for estrogen metabolism. This is one reason why these vegetables are thought to help balance estrogen and progesterone in the body.[35] They've also been associated with cancer prevention. I've continued eating these vegetables daily even after my successful pregnancy because they're so loaded with nutrients. Here are more details about each:

---

[35] Zeligs MA, Diet and estrogen status: the cruciferous connection. J of Medicinal Food 1998 Nov 2; 1: 67-82

Broccoli

I ate broccoli daily or alternated with the next two below. I would use a multicooker (a big pot with a vegetable basket on top) to steam the broccoli. I would put about 1.5" of water at the bottom, boil it and place the basket of broccoli on top – the broccoli was never in the water. I would steam it for about 10 minutes until I could get a fork through it easily but not to the point where much of the color was steamed out. Steaming for too long may destroy some of the nutrients. I found it difficult to eat broccoli raw because it's tough to chew and hard to digest.

You could also consider eating broccoli sprouts. You don't have to eat as much and they actually pack even more nutrients than cooked broccoli. Make sure they're fresh and washed thoroughly. I would eat them raw just by themselves or throw them in a salad.

Brussel Sprouts /Cauliflower

I would cook these similar to the broccoli. I would eat these about every other week with or instead of broccoli just to keep things interesting.

Greens

The types of greens I ate included Collard greens, Kale, Red Chard, Spinach and Mustard Greens. Leafy green vegetables are one of the best kept secrets for women who are trying to enhance fertility and regulate hormones. They are loaded with nutrients and fiber. Kale is a superfood which is great for overall health. It's high in a number of vitamins and minerals which help to detoxify the body. Kale is also a great source of iron and calcium which is important for follicular development. Kale can help reduce inflammation in the body. Collard greens are also a nutritional powerhouse. They are high in fiber and essential nutrients. See the recipe section in this chapter for more on cooking greens.

Carrots & Celery

You can buy these already washed and ready to eat, or you can wash and chop yourself. I would have one serving of each every day. Carrots have phytoestrogens, and celery can act as a natural blood pressure regulator (even though it is high in natural salt). I ate celery throughout my pregnancy and I never had a problem with my blood pressure. Sometimes I would put a little cream cheese on my celery just to give it a little more substance and taste. I also have a soup recipe later in this chapter where you can add these vegetables.

Sweet Potatoes/Yams

Many sources claim that yams can help you conceive twins or you may have heard that sweet potatoes or "yams" are good for fertility. Well, it's very true, the are! First let's clear up the confusion between yams and sweet potatoes. True yams (called Dioscorea) are not the ones you usually find in American grocery stores. They can be found in Africa and Asia and perhaps in some specialized grocery stores in the United States and elsewhere. I've looked for them in my local health food store and they didn't know what I was talking about. In some areas of the world where Dioscorea are readily available, women have a high rate of twins. Although there is not solid research to support the connection between Dioscorea and twins, these yams are thought to stimulate ovulation.

Since regular sweet potatoes or sometimes called "yams" (orange in color) are the most readily available, let's talk about the ways they may benefit fertility. Sweet potatoes are high in vitamin C, B, and vitamin B6. These antioxidants protect against cell damage – your eggs may benefit, no matter how old they are. Sweet potatoes also have an anti-inflammatory affect in the body. They have a positive effect on blood sugar and they are high in fiber which helps to eliminate toxins. Most Americans eat sweet potatoes as part of their Thanksgiving meal, however, they're starting to show up in fast food restaurants as a substitute to the traditional "side of fries". The only problem is that they may be cooked in unhealthy oils. See my recipe later in this chapter to make quick and healthy sweet potato fries.

Onions & Garlic

I would put onions and garlic in everything I could think of. They're great raw or cooked in most recipes. Onions and garlic are a great way to season most dishes because they have so much flavor, you can use less salt and fat. Much has been written about the medicinal qualities of both onions and garlic (and they are also phytoestrogens.) Onions and garlic are in the "allium" family. These are rich in sulfur-containing amino acids and the anti-oxidant quercetin that helps regulate estrogen.[36]

Beans

I realize beans have an image problem because so many people have problems with gas after eating them. Beans are full of antioxidants, fiber, vegetable protein, not to

---

[36] Miodini P, Fioravanti L, Di Fronzo G, Cappelletti V., The two phyto-oestrogens genistein and quercetin exert different effects on oestrogen receptor function., Br J Cancer. 1999 Jun;80(8):1150-5.

mention iron and folic acid. Beans are also phytoestrogens. I had done some reading about how to properly make bean soup to minimize the gas. You need to start with dry beans, do not use canned. Soak them overnight in warm water with a dash of baking soda or lemon juice. In the morning, rinse thoroughly (2-3 times). This helps to soak and rinse out the offensive sugars which cause the bloating and discomfort (there are also dietary supplements you can take which contain food enzymes that assist with the digestion of gas producing foods such as *Beano*). See my bean soup recipe later in this chapter.

Tomatoes and Tomato Salsa

I have included a recipe for tomato salsa at the end of this section, but salsa is naturally low in calories and it contains many healthy vegetables like tomatoes, onions, garlic and peppers. Tomatoes are high in lycopene which can help with conditions like endometriosis.[37] If you don't have time to make your own, the organic store bought varieties are fine and if you read the labels, they are usually free of chemicals and preservatives.

Cucumbers

Cucumbers are high in phytonutrients and lignans and are a source of vitamin C, magnesium, and potassium. They are a high alkaline food (which may make your body sperm friendly) and they are thought to help regulate blood pressure. Cucumbers are over 90% water so they are great for hydration and juicing.

---

[37] Henderson, M. (2008, November 12). Eating tomatoes may help treat endometriosis. Retrieved March 20, 2015, from http://www.livingwithendometriosis.org/2008/11/23/eating-tomatoes-may-help-treat-endometriosis/

Beets

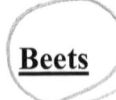

Beets have been associated with increased circulation and improved blood flow throughout the body. They also have benefits related to blood pressure regulation.[38] They are high in antioxidants which can help prevent cell damage.

Salads

An easy way to get more vegetables in your diet is to have a salad every day for lunch and/or dinner. I would have very colorful salads which included: shredded purple cabbage (another cruciferous vegetable), tomatoes, cucumbers, onions, colorful lettuce, beets, olives, avocados, peppers and if you need some protein, you can always throw in some beans, skinless chicken or turkey. You can have the dressing of your choice, but I would pretty much stick with olive oil or coconut oil and red vinegar or balsamic vinegar. Many salad dressings are loaded with sodium, fat and calories, so be sure to read the labels. You can always vary what goes into your salads – just remember, the more colorful, the better. A large salad could account for 2-3 servings of vegetables. Stay away from croutons because they usually contain partially hydrogenated oils. See my salad recipe later in this chapter.

Fruits (three servings a day)

Bananas

Bananas are high in potassium and may help regulate blood pressure. Bananas are also high in iron (which is important

---

[38] Siervo M, Lara J, Ogbonmwan I, Mathers JC., Inorganic nitrate and beetroot juice supplementation reduces blood pressure in adults: a systematic review and meta-analysis, J Nutr. 2013 Jun;143(6):818-26. doi: 10.3945/jn.112.170233. Epub 2013 Apr 17.,

for fertility and during pregnancy) and tryptophan which has a calming effect on the body.

Berries (especially blueberries)

Blueberries are one of the superstars of fruits because they are one of the highest in antioxidants. Antioxidants help to prevent damage by "free radicals" (unstable oxygen molecules) which can be produced by environmental toxins. I would frequently buy them frozen and thaw out one portion every day. I've heard sometimes frozen fruit can actually be fresher than so called "fresh fruit" because it is most likely frozen immediately after it is picked. Non-frozen fruit might actually have been sitting around for a while throughout the distribution process. Additionally, you don't know how long it's been in the supermarket. It can be very frustrating to buy an expensive package of what you think are fresh berries only to get them home and find the bottom layer molded. Other berries I ate included strawberries and blackberries. Try to eat your berries "straight up". Don't add sugar or sugary syrups to them if possible. They're usually very sweet naturally. Berries tend to hold on to quite a few pesticides, so this is one that you would want to buy organic.

Oranges

Oranges are a great source of vitamin C and fiber (vitamin C is an antioxidant and is thought to be good for fertility in women and men – see my section on supplements for more on the benefits of vitamin C for fertility). The vitamin C in oranges may help lengthen menstrual cycles and help with the consistency of cervical mucus. I craved oranges all through the time I was trying to conceive and all throughout my pregnancy.

Kiwis

Kiwis are another great source of vitamin C (even more than oranges)

Red/Purple Grapes & Cherries

Grapes are high in vitamin C and are great for your cardiovascular health. Cherries are high in antioxidants and also have been shown to have anti-inflammatory properties. I would alternate every other week buying grapes and cherries.

Chocolate

If you are looking for a healthy dessert, or if you have an occasional sweet tooth, dark chocolate may be a healthy way to satisfy your cravings with some added benefits. As mentioned in my chapter on preventing miscarriage, chocolate may help prevent pre-eclampsia and dark chocolate is high in antioxidants. I have included a recipe for homemade dark chocolate.

Protein

There may be some evidence that high protein diets such as those recommended in many of the weight loss programs may hurt female fertility. It certainly would be wise to follow a well-balanced diet rather than overloading on protein. Some protein is necessary because the amino acids are essential for men and women to produce quality eggs and sperm. Protein is also needed to help your body manufacture reproductive hormones.

It is recommended to get the majority of your protein from vegetable sources. As reported in the American Journal of Obstetrics and Gynecology, "replacing animal sources of protein, in particular chicken and red meats, with vegetable sources of protein may reduce the risk of infertility due to anovulation."[39]

I did eat meat and poultry, but in very limited amounts. When you eat so many fruits and vegetables a day, you find there's not a lot of room left for heavy meats. Commercially raised meat and poultry contain hormones which act as xenoestrogens. I realize it's hard to completely cut these out of your diet if you're a meat or poultry eater. You can buy organic meats at your health food store, or cut back on the amount you eat (maybe a couple of times per week.) Fish is a great alternative, however recently there's been a lot of press about certain large breeds of fish being contaminated with mercury. I pretty much stuck with Salmon. Salmon is one of the best sources of the Omega-3 fatty acids which are so important to manufacture the good prostaglandins. I found Salmon sold in packets or cans to be the most convenient for sandwiches, salads, etc. and it's been shown to be some of the best in terms of purity.

Soy is another way to get protein in your diet. My local health food store had soy bread which I used to make sandwiches. Soy bread is higher in protein and lower in carbohydrates. It should be refrigerated after purchase. I also had soy nuts which are great to put into a salad or to eat as a snack. Soy can be a hormone regulator because it contains isoflavones which are phytoestrogens. Soy is also a source of essential fatty acids.

---

[39] Chavarro, J. E., Rich-Edwards, J. W., Rosner, B. A., & Willett, W. C. (2008). Protein intake and ovulatory infertility. *American Journal of Obstetrics and Gynecology, 198*(2), 210.e1–210.e7. doi:10.1016/j.ajog.2007.06.057

The Soy Controversy

I should mention that whether or not soy enhances female fertility seems to be an area of controversy. Some sources say soy can actually be detrimental to fertility because the phytoestrogens could act as a contraceptive. However, one study, although done on monkeys (who have menstrual cycles similar to humans), concluded that even though it may lengthen menstrual cycles (which, for me, was a good thing), it did not harm fertility.[40]

Critics of soy mention other reasons it may harm fertility and health including:
- Soy is considered a "goitrogen" which may make it harder for the thyroid to make hormones. However, when studied, this appeared to only be true in populations deficient in iodine.[41]
- Soy is frequently genetically modified (see my "things to avoid" section). When I came up with my fertility diet, less was known or publicized about genetically modified foods. If you do decide to make soy a part of your diet, talk with your local health food store about non GMO soy products.
- Most Americans are consuming unfermented soy which is supposedly worse than the fermented variety. Unfermented soy has phytates which may interfere with nutrient absorption. Some of the most popular unfermented soy products are soymilk, tofu, soy nuts and soy meat alternatives. Fermented soy includes miso, soy sauce, tempeh, and natto.

---

[40] Kaplan, J.R. et al., High isoflavone soy protein does not alter menstrual cyclicity or ovarian function in fully mature, premenopausal monkeys
Fertility and Sterility, Volume 82, S269 - S270

[41] Doerge DR, Sheehan DM., Goitrogenic and estrogenic activity of soy isoflavones, Environ Health Perspect. 2002 Jun;110 Suppl 3:349-53. Review.

So, who do you believe? At the time I was trying to conceive, I did not know the difference between fermented and unfermented soy, but I typically had the unfermented soy because it was easier to incorporate into my diet. The Agency for Healthcare Research and Quality was unable to substantiate claims that soy products (both fermented and unfermented) were harmful or helpful to endocrine function although soy did seem to reduce the incidence of hot flashes.[42]

All controversy aside, I made unfermented soy a regular part of my diet and I have included it here in my pregnancy protocol. I'm a firm believer in eating a variety of foods and not overdoing any one food category. Having said that, soy is typically not recommended for men who are trying to conceive because there does seem to be evidence that the plant estrogens can inhibit sperm production (see my "Just For Men" chapter for more).

DHA Eggs

Eggs are a quick and easy way to get protein in your diet and hard boiled eggs are quite portable. DHA fortified eggs come from chickens fed flax meal and/or have fish oils added to their diet.

Yogurt

There is some evidence that probiotics can promote vaginal health and prevent the overgrowth of harmful organisms.[43]

---

[42] Balk E, Chung M, Chew P, Ip S, Raman G, Kupelnick B, Tatsioni A, Sun Y, Wolk B, DeVine D, Lau J., Effects of Soy on Health Outcomes Agency for Healthcare Research and Quality (US); 2005 Aug. Report No.: 05-E024-2
[43] FEMS Immunol Med Microbiol. 2003 Mar 20;35(2):131-4.

Yogurt can be a good source of beneficial probiotics for a conception friendly environment. It is also a great source of protein and calcium. Look for yogurt with "active or live cultures" on the label. See the fertility yogurt recipe later in this chapter.

Beverages

Soymilk

In addition to the soy I ate in the foods listed above, I would have 16oz of Soymilk many mornings – this was my breakfast along with some fruit. Soymilk can be very filling, so it's great to have as a meal. I would put a little dark chocolate in it for flavor. Again, soymilk is unfermented which has been part of the controversy mentioned earlier.

The Dairy Debate

I've never been a drinker of cow's milk (even as a child), and in terms of fertility, I've read it can be detrimental to ovarian function, especially in older women. Dairy products contain galactose which is a type of sugar found in dairy products (galactose is a component of lactose). Galactose may be harmful to ovarian cells. Populations with higher milk consumption seem to have sharper declines in women's fertility.[44] It was also recently reported that women who consumed low fat dairy were more likely to experience infertility than women who

---

Oral use of Lactobacillus rhamnosus GR-1 and L. fermentum RC-14 significantly alters vaginal flora: randomized, placebo-controlled trial in 64 healthy women.
Reid G[1], Charbonneau D, Erb J, Kochanowski B, Beuerman D, Poehner R, Bruce AW.

[44] Daniel W. Cramer, Huijuan Xu, Timo Sahi, Adult Hypolactasia, Milk Consumption, and Age-specific Fertility, Am. J. Epidemiol. (1994) 139 (3): 282-289.

consumed high fat dairy.[45] I suppose if you're going to consume dairy, you should go for the higher fat version. However, you don't want to be adding a significant amount of fat to your diet so eat in moderation.

While we're talking about dairy, there are some reports that consuming dairy may increase a woman's chances of having multiples.[46] This could be associated with the increased levels of growth hormone in women consuming dairy (coming from the cow's natural growth hormone and synthetic hormones and antibiotics given to cows) which could cause the ovary to release more than one egg. Personally, I find it a bit scary that our milk supply can actually have that effect on a woman. Even though the thought of having twins is quite appealing to anyone trying to conceive, if you're going to consume dairy, I would certainly look for milk which specifically states it is hormone and antibiotic free. Most of the dairy I consumed was in the form of cheese or yogurt. The cheese was usually a small part of a recipe or an ingredient in a restaurant meal.

Vegetable juice

I went through a juicing phase as well. Juicing machines are readily available in most stores that sell kitchen items. This is an easy way to get multitude of vegetables in your diet in a short period of time. You may not get as much fiber, but it still can be very effective. I would juice just about anything. Here are some of the things I would juice (you can add anything here you want – the possibilities are endless):

---

[45] A prospective study of dairy foods intake and anovulatory infertility
Hum. Reprod. (2007) 22 (5): 1340-1347. doi: 10.1093/humrep/dem019 First published online: February 28, 2007
[46] Bakalar, N. (2006, May 30). Rise in Rate of Twin Births May Be Tied to Dairy Case. Retrieved April 3, 2015, from http://www.nytimes.com/2006/05/30/health/30twin.html

Sweet potatoes & Beets – the brighter the better
Parsley
Carrots
Celery
Cucumbers

Occasionally, I would throw in some fruits (like grapes & apples) to sweeten things up a bit. If you buy a juicing machine, most come with a recipe book. I didn't follow a recipe, I just made sure to juice a wide variety of fruits and vegetables each week.

In addition to my own juicing, I would have store bought canned vegetable juice sometime in the afternoon. Some of these can be quite high in sodium, so look for a low-sodium variety. I'm not a big advocate of canned products, because the cans are frequently lined in plastic (which is one of my substances to avoid). So I would only buy and drink canned vegetables and/or juice in moderation.

Another note about convenience: I would only juice once per week, but I would juice enough to have one serving every day. Store the juice covered in the refrigerator. I would actually break up my juice in glasses (individual servings – about 8 oz. each) so I could just grab one when I was ready. Be sure to stir before drinking because much of the beneficial sediment falls to the bottom of the glass when it's made ahead of time.

Wheatgrass

Wheatgrass has recently gained in popularity and is showing up in juice bars everywhere. When I think of wheatgrass, I think of cows grazing in a pasture, but it's a

great food for people too. So why is wheatgrass so good for fertility? Here are some reasons:
- It is a high alkaline food. You need a balanced pH level so that your body is sperm friendly. If you are not familiar with pH, it ranges between 1-14 with 7 being neutral. If your body is under 7, it may be too acidic. Ideally, your pH would be a bit on the alkaline side in the 7.35—7.45 range.[47] An alkaline environment is best for conception.
- Wheatgrass also contains folic acid. Folic acid has been found to prevent neural tube defects and it's recommended that women who are trying to conceive take folic acid before they try to get pregnant.
- Wheatgrass enhances men's fertility because it is high in antioxidants. Sperm are actually very fragile creatures. Men who have a diet high in antioxidants can protect their sperm from free radical damage due to environmental factors.
- Wheatgrass is thought to purify the blood, liver and kidneys for detoxification.

There are also external ways to use wheatgrass, for example, did you know you could bathe in it? As odd as that sounds, you can add some wheatgrass juice to your bath water and soak for 1/2 hour. This is thought to disinfect the skin and it is actually reported to increase your red blood cells. It is also great if you have itchy skin or body odor.

Spirulina

Spirulina is a chlorophyll dense plant that grows in the wild, but commercially available. Spirulina is grown in a

---

[47] Schwalfenberg, G. K. (2012). The Alkaline Diet: Is There Evidence That an Alkaline pH Diet Benefits Health? Journal of Environmental and Public Health, 2012, 727630. doi:10.1155/2012/727630

controlled environment to ensure that pollutants do not contaminate the product. When spirulina is harvested it is laid to dry before being crushed into flakes or powder. Flakes can be easily added to salads or sauces, while the powder can be mixed with water or in shakes. The benefits include:

- It is a protein rich food which is needed for hormone production and high egg quality.
- It is high in the beneficial omega 3's which not only help with hormone production, but they also have an overall anti-inflammatory effect on the body.
- It has chlorophyll which helps to detoxify. It can bind with heavy metals to remove them.
- It is high in iron which has been shown to help with fertility and is very important should you become pregnant.
- It is high in B vitamins including folic acid.
- It is high in calcium which is important for pregnancy (it can have 26 times the amount of calcium in milk!).

At the end of this chapter I have a recipe for a spirulina (or wheatgrass) smoothie.

Water, Water, Water

I know there have been some stories in the media about how it's a myth that you need 8 glasses of water a day – I don't believe it and neither do plenty of experts who say just the opposite. Much has been written about the critical role water plays in almost all bodily functions and I think it was an essential piece of my successful pregnancy. Water helps to keep your bowels regular. You don't want toxic substances building up in your system by getting constipated (eating fruits and vegetables will help with this too). If you're dehydrated, your cervical/vaginal fluids will not be the right consistency for sperm to swim upstream.

Your fallopian tubes need to be properly lubricated for the egg to travel down. It just makes sense if you don't have enough hydration, *everything* is going to be dried out. You want to get in the habit of drinking lots of water now because you'll want to continue this when you're pregnant. When I was pregnant I drank between 64-80oz of water per day and I always had a good volume of amniotic fluid (there is a special test they do to measure amniotic fluid – it looks somewhat like an ultrasound machine). The nurse would always say "I'll bet you drink a lot of water" because my test results always looked good.

In Ayurvedic medicine, there is a practice of drinking water the first thing in the morning on an empty stomach called "Usha Paana Chikitsa". This is thought to help cleanse the colon and purify the blood. The body is better able to absorb nutrients after this process. This is thought to help with a number of conditions including infertility. You should not consume alcoholic beverages the night before and you should not eat anything for one hour after drinking the water. Sources on this recommend 5-6 glasses of water upon waking, however, I am hesitant to recommend this amount all at once since too much water too quickly can overload your kidneys. I frequently did (and still do) drink a couple of glasses of water first thing in the morning.

Bottled vs. Tap?

I frequently have wondered which was better – bottled vs. tap water. This is another area where there is quite a bit of conflicting information. It probably depends on where in the country you live, the condition of the pipes in your home, the source of the bottled water, etc. I had read that there was a higher miscarriage rate in women who drank tap water during their pregnancies. Fluoride which is added to tap water has been associated with declining birth rates[48] and has also been associated with hypothyroidism.[49] Even arsenic and pharmaceutical drugs have been detected in tap water…yikes! If you want to drink tap water, perhaps you should have it tested. Buy a good filter and change it frequently. Be extra careful if you drink well water. As I mention later in the "Preventing Miscarriage" chapter, well water may be a source of nitrites which should be avoided. For all these reasons, I drank bottled water. I did some research on local suppliers of bottled water to make sure they had a good filtration system. You should also look for a fluoride free variety.

Tea & Herbs

Although scientific research on herbs and herbal teas is limited, I researched a number of sources on herbal remedies which can help fertility. The teas I drank included:
- Red Raspberry which is reported to tone the uterus and pelvic muscles
- Chasteberry (Vitex) is supposed to have a positive effect on your FSH by increasing LH (and thereby decreasing FSH). Chasteberry is also thought to help if a woman has high prolactin levels.
- Dong Quai can help increase menstrual flow in women who have very light periods. It can also help with short periods and irregular cycles.

---

[48] Freni SC, Exposure to high fluoride concentrations in drinking water is associated with decreased birth rates, J Toxicol Environ Health. 1994 May;42(1):109-21.
[49] S Peckham, D Lowery, S Spencer, Are fluoride levels in drinking water associated with hypothyroidism prevalence in England? A large observational study of GP practice data and fluoride levels in drinking water, J Epidemiol Community Health doi:10.1136/jech-2014-204971

My Specific Pregnancy Protocol

- Red Clover may help regulate your cycles. It has phytoestrogens and can help with your body's pH which can make cervical mucus more sperm friendly.
- Green Tea – Some sources draw a correlation between drinking green tea and increased rates of conception, although this could possibly be attributed to green tea drinkers having healthier lifestyles. One widely cited study in The American Journal of Public Health reported that drinking 1½ cups or more of tea daily can double the odds of conception per cycle.[50] However, this study did not specify what kind of tea the participants drank. Regular tea and green tea both have polyphenols and hypoxanthine which may be responsible for more viable embryos and possibly a greater chance of fertilization. Although green tea has caffeine, it is found in lesser amounts than other caffeinated beverages (but I would recommend drinking decaffeinated). On the downside, in pregnancy, some sources claim green tea may possibly increase the chance of pregnancy loss because the tannins could have a negative effect on a developing embryo by constricting blood vessel formation (although I was unable to find scientific research to support an association between green tea and pregnancy loss). The tannins may also interfere with iron absorption. Since green tea has a number of health benefits unrelated to fertility, I included it in my diet. I drank mint flavored decaffeinated green tea when I was experiencing morning sickness after I conceived my daughter (this was before I knew of any possible association with miscarriage), but obviously it didn't hurt my pregnancy.

---

[50] B Caan, C P Quesenberry, Jr, and A O Coates, Differences in fertility associated with caffeinated beverage consumption, Am J Public Health. 1998 February; 88(2): 270–274.

I brewed these teas together and consumed them in the first half of my menstrual cycle only (up through day 14). My logic here was I wanted to have a totally pure system when I conceived. I had at least two cups per day. I have included a recipe for "fertility tea" at the end of this chapter and there are many fertility blends on the market now which were not available when I was trying to conceive.

Aside from the teas I drank, I did not go the herbal route. I know there are many good herbalists out there who can guide you through the multitude of herbal remedies that are available. I know herbal remedies are considered natural, however many herbs can actually be toxic if they're not taken properly. Additionally, I did not want to rely on another paid professional to help me weed through all the options in addition to buying what might be expensive herbal concoctions. In no way am I saying herbal remedies aren't legitimate; my point here is to tell you what steps I took that proved to be successful.

Coffee/Caffeine

Caffeine is thought disrupt reproductive hormones and women may be more sensitive to its affects. One study found: "moderate consumption of caffeine was associated with reduced estradiol concentrations among white women, whereas caffeinated soda and green tea intakes were associated with increased estradiol concentrations among all races."[51] When pregnant, caffeine can cross the placenta (see more in my chapter on preventing miscarriage). In terms of trying to conceive, caffeine should be reduced or cut out of your diet. If at all possible,

---

[51] Karen C Schliep, Enrique F Schisterman, Sunni L Mumford, Anna Z Pollack, Cuilin Zhang, Aijun Ye, Joseph B Stanford, Ahmad O Hammoud, Christina A Porucznik, and Jean Wactawski-Wende, Caffeinated beverage intake and reproductive hormones among premenopausal women in the BioCycle Study, Am J Clin Nutr. 2012 Feb; 95(2): 488–497.

try to replace regular coffee with the decaffeinated variety or the teas mentioned above.

Carbohydrates

Watch out for those "bad" carbohydrates. I'm sure you've already heard that you should avoid many of the processed "white foods". These foods break down easily and raise blood sugar. This raises insulin levels which could increase the level of male hormones produced by the ovary. This ultimately could result in ovulation irregularities. One study found: "total carbohydrate intake and dietary glycemic load were positively related to ovulatory infertility".[52] On the other hand, "good" carbohydrates are digested more slowly. These include darker breads, beans and vegetables. The glycemic index ranks foods based on how they affect blood sugar or glucose. Foods that are high on the glycemic index quickly raise blood sugar and insulin.

So what type of carbs should you be eating?
Here is a guide with some common foods from the American Diabetes Association[53] (GI stands for glycemic index and the lower, the better):

Low GI Foods (55 or less)

100% stone-ground whole wheat or pumpernickel bread
Oatmeal (rolled or steel-cut), oat bran, muesli
Pasta, converted rice, barley, bulgar

---

[52] AChavarro, J. E., Rich-Edwards, J. W., Rosner, B. A., & Willett, W. C. (2009). A prospective study of dietary carbohydrate quantity and quality in relation to risk of ovulatory infertility. European Journal of Clinical Nutrition, 63(1), 78–86. doi:10.1038/sj.ejcn.1602904

[53] Glycemic Index and Diabetes. (2014, May 14). Retrieved March 7, 2015, from http://www.diabetes.org/food-and-fitness/food/what-can-i-eat/understanding-carbohydrates/glycemic-index-and-diabetes.html

Sweet potato, corn, yam, lima/butter beans, peas, legumes and lentils
Most fruits, non-starchy vegetables and carrots

Medium GI Foods (56-69)

Whole wheat, rye and pita bread
Quick oats
Brown, wild or basmati rice, couscous

High GI Foods (70 or more)

White bread or bagel
Corn flakes, puffed rice, bran flakes, instant oatmeal
Shortgrain white rice, rice pasta, mac-n-cheese from mix
Russet potato, pumpkin
Pretzels, rice cakes, popcorn, saltine crackers
Melons and pineapple

When I was trying to conceive, the vast majority of my carbohydrates came from the low glycemic category and I think you'll find that most foods I recommend are as well.

Do you have to be perfect with your diet?

I certainly wasn't perfect, but I ate well *most* of the time. Twice a week (Friday and Saturday nights) my husband and I would go out to dinner. On these nights, I ate anything I wanted. That's only 2 meals per week, but going a little crazy a couple nights really helped me stick to a healthy diet the rest of the time. On week nights, when my husband was home for dinner, I would make a regular dinner (pasta, casseroles, etc.), but I would make these meals as healthy as possible making sure they didn't have a lot of fat, hydrogenated oils, etc. I would be sure to get all my servings of fruits and vegetables in before the evening meal and whenever possible, I would include vegetables as part of the evening meal.

Recipes

Although I am not the kind of cook who follows recipes very closely (I usually look up 2-3 recipes and combine the parts I like of each), I have included some of my favorites below.

Sweet Potato Fries

1. Take a medium sweet potato, leave the skin on
2. Wash thoroughly with a white vinegar spray
3. Slice with a grid shape french-fry slicer or cut into fry size pieces
4. Lay the pieces onto a baking sheet and try not to overlap
5. Drizzle with olive oil and season with salt, pepper or other seasonings as desired
6. Bake for about 18-25 minutes until potatoes are soft and/or crispy depending on your preference
7. Be sure to flip the potatoes over after the first 10 -15 minutes for even cooking

Baked Cruciferous Vegetables

Earlier, I mentioned lightly steaming these vegetables to preserve their nutrition. If you prefer to bake them, here are instructions:
1. Cut a head of broccoli or cauliflower so the flowery part of the vegetable is in pieces about 1 inch wide (for brussel sprouts, cut in half) You can also include the stems which have nutritional value as well
2. Place in large bowl
3. Chop finely 1-2 cloves of garlic and mix in
4. Drizzle with olive oil and season with sea salt or other seasonings of your choice and stir so all pieces are evenly coated

5. Spread vegetables out on a baking sheet and try not to overlap.
6. Bake at 400 for about 15 minutes.

Fertility Tea Recipe

1. Chasteberry-Vitex
2. Green Tea (preferably decaffeinated)
3. Red Raspberry Leaf
4. Red Clover
5. Dong Quai

When you are ready to brew your tea, you can do it a couple of ways:

1. If you are using tea bags (pre-packaged tea), you can get a large tea brewing container and add all the teabags and brew together. If the teas have different brewing times on the package, use the one with the shortest brewing time. Once the tea is brewed, store it in the refrigerator and heat one cup at a time (or you can drink it iced). If it is too concentrated, you can dilute it down with a bit with water.
2. If you are using loose tea, combine equal parts of the loose teas together in a bowl (then store in a glass container). When you are ready to have a cup of tea, get a tea ball and use about 1-2 teaspoons of the mixture per cup (6-8 oz). Use fresh water in a teapot (if you are concerned about your water quality, use bottled water) and boil to about 170-180 degrees. Close the tea ball and place in the cup and put your heated water in the cup with the tea ball. If you would like to make a pitcher of tea, you can use a "tea sock" which will hold much more tea. Place the pitcher in the refrigerator after it is brewed to have later. It is usually recommended to drink within 72 hours for maximum freshness.

Fertility Salad Recipe

1. Take one head of red (purple) cabbage. Cut it in half and save the rest for later. Shred about 1 cup with a cheese shredder as finely as possible. Raw cabbage can be a little hard to digest, so if it is shredded finely, it will help.
2. Cut up about 1/3 of a large cucumber
3. Peel a ripe avocado, cut in half and discard the pit. Chop ½ of the avocado and save the rest for later.
4. Cut a tomato in half and cut into cube size pieces.
5. Add about 1 tablespoon of extra virgin olive oil
6. Add some balsamic vinegar if desired
7. Add salt and pepper to taste

Greens For Fertility

1. Get a bundle of greens (Kale, Collard, etc.) and thoroughly wash with a white vinegar spray
2. Cut greens down into bite size pieces in a crisscross fashion
3. Heat some olive oil (start with a couple of tablespoons) in a pan using moderate heat as olive oil has a low burning point
4. Put the greens in the hot pan, (it is okay if they still have some moisture as this will help with the cooking) sprinkle with garlic salt, pepper or any other seasonings you desire
5. Chop about ½ onion and a clove of garlic and fry in the pan with the greens
6. Cook for about 8-10 minutes while continually flipping the greens over for even cooking. Your plan will be overflowing, but the greens will cook down in a few minutes.

Hearty Bean, Vegetable and Barley Soup

1. Get a 1 pound bag of dried organic red beans, black beans or a mixture (darker beans are higher in antioxidants).
2. Soak the beans overnight in warm water with about a teaspoon of baking soda in a large bowl
3. The next morning, rinse the beans thoroughly 2-3 times
4. Fill a large pot ¾ full with a mixture of water and vegetable or beef broth and bring to a boil
5. Add beans
6. Chop and add: 1 large onion, 4-5 stalks of celery, 4-5 large carrots, 1 russet potato, a couple cloves of garlic
7. Add 1/3 cup dried barley
8. Add ½ lb of chopped ham if desired
9. Add seasonings (1 tsp salt, 1 tsp pepper, sprinkle with chili powder or mesquite seasoning if desired)
10. Constantly stir soup for at least 2 hours until it thickens up
11. When beans are soft, remove about 2 cups of the soup mixture and mash with a hand mixer then return it to the pot. This will thicken the soup even further.
12. You can add some soup noodles 15 minutes prior to serving, but usually the barley took the place of noodles in my soup.

This recipe makes a large pot of soup. Freeze leftovers in individual portions for a quick and healthy meal.

Fertility Yogurt Recipe

Yogurt can be a fertility enhancing food because it has protein which is good for hormone development, and it is a good source of probiotics which can promote vaginal health and the proper environment for conception (look for "live

cultures" on the label.) The blueberries in this recipe are loaded with antioxidants which help egg quality and the nuts are great source of the good fats.
1. Start with plain unsweetened yogurt. Full fat dairy was found in one study to be good for female fertility - so you can choose full fat yogurt if desired. Greek yogurt is highest in protein.
2. Sweeten yogurt with some liquid stevia. Artificial sweeteners like aspartame may have some detrimental effects on your health. Stevia is a safe alternative. Use a couple of squirts from the dropper to taste.
3. Add about 1/3 cup of raw walnuts and almonds. Be sure to get the refrigerated ones at your health food store. As mentioned earlier, when nuts are roasted, it destroys their natural oils.
4. Add a handful of frozen organic blueberries. You can also use fresh blueberries but adding frozen ones actually makes the yogurt taste like ice cream.
5. Stir it up and add a tiny bit of sugar sprinkled lightly on the top if you desire.

Spirulina or Wheatgrass Smoothie

1. 1 cup of milk (preferably almond, coconut, or soy) or 1 cup of water, cold green tea, cold fertility tea, apple juice or other fruit juice of your choice
2. 1 cup of fresh or frozen mixed berries, or other fruit of your choice
3. 1 fresh or frozen banana
4. 2 teaspoons of spirulina or wheatgrass powder
5. A little honey, maple syrup, or stevia to sweeten (optional)
6. ice as needed
7. Mix in a blender until smooth

Variations include adding yogurt, supplemental probiotics, granulated bee pollen and vitamins. It is not recommended to use hot liquids as they may neutralize the enzymes.

Egg Salad or Salmon Salad Sandwich

1. Chop 1-2 DHA fortified hard boiled eggs
2. Chop ¼ cup organic celery
3. Shred 1 small carrot
4. Chop 1 sweet pickle (or use 1-2 tablespoons of sweet relish)
5. 1-2 tablespoons of organic mayonnaise or salad dressing
6. Mix all ingredients together and serve on whole grain bread or soy bread

For salmon salad, substitute one packet of fresh water salmon for the eggs or salmon can be added to the egg recipe.

Avocado Sandwich

1. ½ ripe avocado, peeled, with pit removed
2. ½ ripe tomato sliced
3. 1 leaf lettuce

Slice avocado and season with some garlic salt or garlic powder if desired. Layer avocado, tomato and lettuce on whole grain bread or soy bread, add organic mayonnaise.

Tomato Salsa

Chop finely:
1. 2-3 ripe tomatoes (variety of your choice)
2. 1/3 cup onion
3. 1 clove garlic
4. 1-2 sprigs of cilantro
5. 1-2 jalapeno peppers (or other peppers of your choice)
6. Add a few drops of olive oil
7. Mix together and eat with whole grain chips

One trick I learned to cut down on carbohydrates is to snap each chip in half and load each half up with salsa. This avoids "double dipping" if you're sharing with others and you'll consume only half the carbohydrates and calories.

Healthy Guacamole

1. Peel 2-3 ripe avocados, remove pit, chop and mash in a small bowl
2. Add 1-2 tablespoons salsa (either from the recipe above or from a jar)
3. Sprinkle with garlic powder to taste
4. Sprinkle with seasoning salt to taste
5. If desired, chop 1/3 cup lettuce and a small tomato and add to bowl
6. Mix together well and serve with whole grain chips

Healthy Dark Chocolate recipe

1. ⅓ cup organic cocoa powder
2. ½ cup coconut oil or ¾ cup of butter/margarine substitute (such as omega 3 buttery spread)
3. 2 tablespoons honey (variations include agave, liquid stevia to taste, maple syrup)
4. ½ teaspoon vanilla
5. dash of salt
6. Water or milk as needed for consistency

In a double boiler, melt cocoa powder, butter substitute, sugar, milk, sweetener and water/milk as needed. Mix all ingredients well. Pour into an ice tray for individual servings. If desired, add some almonds and walnuts in the ice tray before pouring chocolate. Put in freezer until firm and remove the individual pieces from the tray. Store in the refrigerator to maintain freshness.

My Pregnancy Protocol - Part II
Supplements

Natural Progesterone Cream

Another piece of the equation when dealing with estrogen dominance is your progesterone level. Progesterone opposes the effect of estrogen. I knew my progesterone was low from one of the blood tests I had done during my fertility treatments. Also, my menstrual cycles were quite short (indicating my progesterone was falling too quickly after ovulation.) I kept coming across natural progesterone cream in my reading which I immediately began using. Natural progesterone is a plant extract which has a molecular structure identical to the progesterone produced by your body (unlike the synthetic progesterone widely used by the medical community). Using natural progesterone and avoiding xenoestrogens can put your hormones back in balance. Since my menstrual cycles were as short as 21 days (they would range between 21-24 days when I first started trying to get pregnant), I knew progesterone cream could help maintain my uterine lining and lengthen my menstrual cycle.

Natural progesterone cream is used between days 12-27 of your menstrual cycle (if it goes that long) and you can purchase it over the counter at health food stores. You can also purchase it on-line, but I prefer to buy products carried by my health food store because I know they enforce a high quality standard with the manufacturers. Follow the directions on the package. The label will tell you how much to use and how many times per day. Be sure to put it on different parts of your body with each application so your skin doesn't build up resistance. There are different brands on the market, you just need to look for at least 480mg of USP progesterone per oz. The symbol 'USP' stands for United States Pharmacopeia. If a product has this symbol, it must meet certain quality standards so you can be assured you are getting the amount of progesterone stated on the package label.

I should mention that there seems to be differing opinions in the medical community about natural progesterone cream (assuming they've even heard of it). Some doctors don't think you can get enough to do any good through a topical application. However, there are other doctors who think just the opposite --- that progesterone is best absorbed through the skin. There are even doctors who feel you can get too much with continued use! All I can tell you is *my* experience. I was fairly certain from previous lab work that I was progesterone deficient in the second half of my cycle. My menstrual cycles did lengthen in the months before I conceived, frequently 26 - 28 days. Most importantly, I did conceive while using it.

Many manufacturers of natural progesterone cream claim that it can help prevent first trimester miscarriage by giving your body the progesterone support it needs. Even though I had a problem with miscarriage, I did not use it during pregnancy. I used it up until the time I found out I was pregnant. When you do become pregnant, talk to your doctor about whether it's safe to continue using natural progesterone cream.

Natural Ways To Increase Progesterone

If you are following my pregnancy protocol and eating from my fertility diet, most of the following foods should already be incorporated, but here are a few of the specific ways you can increase progesterone naturally:

1. Unroasted nuts like almonds/walnuts and seeds like sunflower seeds can help your body increase progesterone naturally. You should look for them in the refrigerated section of your health food store.
2. Vitamin B6, vitamin C
3. Avocados – These are an excellent source of plant sterols. Plant sterols help to create a balance between estrogen and progesterone which will help with estrogen dominance.
4. Leafy Green Vegetables – These contain magnesium which will help your body manufacture progesterone naturally.
5. Protein – Hormones are essentially proteins, so eat organic meats in moderation, or vegetable protein as mentioned earlier.
6. In addition to magnesium in foods, take magnesium as a supplement (see more below).

Multivitamin

It's a jungle out there when it comes to vitamins. I didn't like the idea of taking a handful of vitamins every day. Most of the vitamins I have included in my pregnancy protocol are available in the amounts recommended through a high quality multivitamin. If you are following my fertility diet, you will get a large portion of your daily requirements through your diet as well. I took one multivitamin a day (the kind you can buy at a health food store that ensures quality and purity).

Make sure your multivitamin contains the following:

Selenium

Selenium has been found in large healthy follicles[54] and it has been associated with a decreased risk of miscarriage (see more in my preventing miscarriage chapter).

Iron

It was found that women who consume iron supplements and non-heme iron from other sources may decrease the risk of ovulatory infertility.[55] Plants and iron-fortified foods contain non-heme iron only, whereas meat, seafood, and poultry contain both heme and non-heme iron. Heme iron is more bioavailable than non-heme iron[56] which means that it is more easily absorbed. The daily recommended amount of iron for women is 18mg.

Vitamin D

The European Society of Endocrinology reported that vitamin D can improve reproductive hormone production in women and help women with PCOS with menstrual frequency. In men, vitamin D can help with semen quality and testosterone levels.[57] Most people don't get enough vitamin D from sunlight especially now that there's been so much attention put on preventing skin cancer. Interestingly, I've read that to get adequate vitamin D from the sun, you actually need to be out during the hours we're

---

[54] M. J. Ceko, K. Hummitzsch, N. Hatzirodos, W. M. Bonner, J. B. Aitken, D. L. Russell, M. Lane, R. J. Rodgers H. H. Harris
X-Ray fluorescence imaging and other analyses identify selenium and GPX1 as important in female reproductive function, Metallomics, 2015, 7, 71-82
DOI: 10.1039/C4MT00228H

[55] Chavarro JW, Rich-Edwards,JW, Rosner BA, Willett WC.
Iron intake and risk of ovulatory infertility, Obstet Gynecol. 2006 Nov;108(5):1145-52.

[56] Iron Dietary Supplement Fact Sheet. (2015, February 19). Retrieved April 13, 2015, from http://ods.od.nih.gov/factsheets/Iron-HealthProfessional/

[57] Elisabeth Lerchbaum, and Barbara R Obermayer-Pietsch, Vitamin D and fertility-a systematic review, Eur J Endocrinol January 24, 2012 EJE-11-0984

usually told to avoid (i.e. 10:00am – 2:00pm). The recommended amount for a supplement is usually 600IU.

Vitamin C

Vitamin C may help with luteal phase defect[58] (where hormones are insufficient in the second half of the menstrual cycle) and it may improve the consistency of cervical mucus.

B Vitamins

Our bodies produce a substance called "homocysteine" from the digestion of protein. High levels of homocysteine may contribute to miscarriage and pregnancy complications.[59] Vitamin B12, B6 and B9 (also known as folic acid) can help keep homocysteine levels in check.

Inositol (or myo-inositol) is another one of the B complex vitamins and it has been found in the follicular fluid of higher quality eggs.[60] It is frequently found in some supplements but it's something you should look for in your multivitamin. Animal studies have shown that myo-inositol helps with blastocyst development. Myo-inositol is especially helpful for women with PCOS[61], but other women may find it helpful as well. It is thought to increase

---

[58] Henmi H et al. Effects of ascorbic acid supplementation on serum progesterone levels in patients with a luteal phase defect. Fertility and Sterility August 2003; 80:459-461.

[59] Del Bianco A, Maruotti G, Fulgieri AM, Celeste T, Lombardi L, Amato NA, Pietropaolo F. Recurrent spontaneous miscarriages and hyperhomocysteinemia Minerva Ginecol. 2004 Oct;56(5):379-83.

[60] Tony T.Y. Chiu, Michael S. Rogers, Eric L.K. Law, Christine M. Briton-Jones, L.P. Cheung, Christopher J. Haines, Follicular fluid and serum concentrations of myo-inositol in patients undergoing IVF: relationship with oocyte quality, Hum. Reprod. (2002) 17 (6): 1591-1596. doi: 10.1093/humrep/17.6.1591

[61] Enrico Papaleo, Vittorio Unfer, Jean-Patrice Baillargeon, Lucia De Santis, Francesco Fusi, Claudio Brigante, Guido Marelli, Ilaria Cino, Anna Redaelli, and Augusto Ferrari, Myo-inositol in patients with polycystic ovary syndrome: a novel method for ovulation induction. Gynecological Endocrinology 23(12):700 (2007) PMID 17952759

insulin sensitivity of the ovary which helps egg quality. It is recommended that a woman who is trying to conceive should take it three months before they get pregnant while their eggs are forming in their ovary.

Vitamin A (use with caution)

Be careful with Vitamin A because too much can cause birth defects in a developing fetus. Some manufacturers of prenatal vitamins have actually taken the Vitamin A completely out. If you're consuming many of the colorful fruits and vegetables and taking a multivitamin, you'll probably be getting an adequate and safe amount of Vitamin A.

You may also need to take additional amounts of these in addition to the multivitamin:

Folic Acid

I took 400mcg of folic acid (My multivitamin also had 400mcg of folic acid – so I was taking a total of 800mcg of folic acid). Folic acid has been proven to reduce the chance of neural tube birth defects and there may be evidence that it might help prevent Down Syndrome. You need to take it before you get pregnant to reap these benefits, so now is the right time to start. After you get pregnant, you should continue taking folic acid (even if it's part of your prenatal vitamins) since it has also been associated with a decreased risk of miscarriage. Folic acid has an added bonus of being good for your cardiovascular health.

Calcium-Magnesium

I took 1000mg of calcium citrate (this absorbs better than calcium carbonate) along with magnesium in one supplement. I continued taking calcium after I was pregnant because it has also been associated with blood pressure regulation[62] which is very important during pregnancy (see blood pressure below). You can also get calcium through your diet, for instance, my soymilk was calcium fortified and yogurt is another great source. Many vegetables in my fertility diet are also high in calcium.

Magnesium supplementation has been shown to help previously infertile women succeed in getting pregnant. The women in one study received supplemental magnesium which normalized their red cell magnesium levels and helped with fertility.[63] My fertility diet has many foods high in magnesium, but the calcium supplement I took (the 1000mg mentioned above) was a cal-mag combination. Magnesium is also supposed to help with calcium absorption and regulation. The recommended amount for women between the ages of 31-50 is 320mg.

Vitamin E

I took 400IU of Vitamin E (mixed tocopherals). I've heard Vitamin E called "vitamin everything" because it's so good for your health. It can also act as a hormone regulator. One study found "Vitamin E administration may improve the endometrial response in unexplained infertile women via the likely antioxidant and the anticoagulant effects".[64]

---

[62] Karppanen H., Minerals and blood pressure, Ann Med. 1991 Aug;23(3):299-305.
[63] Howard JM, Davies S, Hunniset, A, Red cell magnesium and glutathione peroxidase in infertile women--effects of oral supplementation with magnesium and selenium, Magnes Res. 1994 Mar;7(1):49-57.
[64] Vitamin E effect on controlled ovarian stimulation of unexplained infertile women. Cicek N, Eryilmaz OG, Sarikaya E, Gulerman C, Genc Y.
J Assist Reprod Genet. 2012 Apr;29(4):325-8. doi: 10.1007/s10815-012-9714-1.

Omega-3 fatty acids

As mentioned previously, these fats help your body manufacture hormones and shift the balance in favor of the "good" prostaglandins. You can get these through your diet, but a supplement can be helpful as well. According to the DHA EPA Omega-3 Institute and The Dieticians of North America, the recommended dosage is 500mg of DHA EPA.[65] Check with your health food store for information on purity of fish oil. As I have mentioned previously, many fish have contaminants and this can transfer to fish oils as well.

More Optional Supplements

Evening Primrose Oil

I actually did not take Evening Primrose Oil (EPO) as an oral supplement (but it was an ingredient in my natural progesterone cream). I have come across EPO frequently in my research so I wanted to include it here. It comes from a wildflower which grows in North America (the oil is extracted from the seeds.) You can take this supplement in in capsules or liquid form. It should be kept in the refrigerator and out of sunlight.

Evening Primrose Oil is high in vitamin E and GLA (gamma-linoleic acid) which helps your body manufacture the "good" prostaglandins which I explained earlier. GLA works as a vessel dilator and blood thinner.

Evening primrose oil is also thought to improve the uterine lining and strengthen the placenta. It acts as an anti-

---

[65] WHat is the recommended intake of DHA EPA per day? (n.d.). Retrieved March 12, 2015, from http://www.dhaomega3.org/FAQ/WHat-is-the-recommended-intake-of-DHA EPA-per-day

inflammatory which can help with conditions like endometriosis and pelvic inflammatory disorders.

If you are having problems with the quality of your cervical mucus, Evening Primrose Oil may help with this as well. If you are experiencing thick or hostile cervical mucus, it may help you attain the "egg white" consistency that is necessary to help sperm swim. It is recommended not to use this supplement during the last half of the menstrual cycle (luteal phase) since it may cause uterine contractions. This could make conception less likely since it may be harder for the egg to implant.

It should be noted that some studies have questioned its effectiveness as a fertility enhancer, however this could be attributed to poor study design.

DHEA

DHEA is not to be confused with DHA which can also be important for fertility as mentioned earlier. DHEA is talked about in the literature as a supplement to use to improve egg quality. I did not know about DHEA when I was trying to conceive, but I thought it was worth mentioning it here since studies seem to support its effectiveness. It is a steroid hormone which is produced by your adrenal gland. It is usually at its highest around the age of 30 and declines as we get older. DHEA is a precursor to hormone production and is eventually converted to hormones like estrogen and testosterone. Around the age of menopause, women not only lack estrogens but also androgens. As reported by the National Institutes of Health on a study of women undergoing IVF: "Our results show that DHEA supplementation improves the ovarian function in poor responders and in women over 40 years, suggesting that this molecule alone can raise fecundity and fertility treatment success in women with poor prognosis for pregnancy."[66]

There are differing opinions about taking DHEA as a supplement. First, you should check with your doctor and have hormonal levels checked. DHEA can interact with some medications and it can raise hormone levels which can be problematic if you have had, or are at high risk for, some hormone dependent cancers. The women in the study (undergoing IVF) received three tablets daily of 25 mg micronized DHEA for at least 12 weeks before starting a long stimulation protocol for IVF.

Baby Aspirin

I took one per day (81mg). When I went through fertility treatments, baby aspirin was part of the protocol. It may increase the circulation to the uterus (thereby building up the uterine lining) and the ovaries. I decided I would continue with the baby aspirin even though I wasn't going through fertility treatments anymore. I figured the dose was so low it probably wouldn't hurt anything and it just may help. One thing I did notice in the months before my successful pregnancy is my periods were a little heavier (although still light by most people's standards). In the years prior to my successful pregnancy, my periods were very scanty. Sometimes I would totally forget it was that time of the month – and I never had an accident. I almost thought I was going through menopause because my menstrual flow was so light. Perhaps the baby aspirin helped with my uterine lining enough to support a healthy attachment. This is the only "medication" I took on my

---

[66] Fusi FM, Ferrario M, Bosisio C, Arnoldi M, Zanga L., DHEA supplementation positively affects spontaneous pregnancies in women with diminished ovarian function. Gynecol Endocrinol. 2013 Oct;29(10):940-3. doi: 10.3109/09513590.2013.819087. Epub 2013 Jul 26.

natural journey to a successful pregnancy. Talk to your doctor before taking aspirin because there may be contraindications (i.e. clotting problems, allergies, other medications or even vitamins you may be taking). Once I had a positive pregnancy test, I discontinued the baby aspirin. Again, I wanted a totally pure system for my pregnancy.

As far as miscarriage, a recent study failed to demonstrate that aspirin is effective in preventing pregnancy loss, although it did seem to help women get pregnant after a previous miscarriage. It was reported, "women who had experienced a single, recent pregnancy loss (before 4 1/2 months of pregnancy and within the past year) had an increased rate of pregnancy and live birth while on aspirin therapy"[67]. Again, I discontinued taking aspirin once I got pregnant.

Bee Pollen, Royal Jelly, Bee Propolis

Bee pollen contains almost all the nutrients that humans need. You may be thinking that bee pollen and royal jelly are strange things for humans to consume. Bee pollen is about 40% protein in the form of free amino acids and is easily used by the body. Hormones are made of proteins and bee pollen is a great source as is royal jelly. Royal jelly also contains vitamin D, E, iron, calcium and acetylcholine which can help with nerve transmission from cell to cell. The queen bee is exclusively fed royal jelly helping her lay thousands of eggs per day.

Although scientific research is limited on bee products and fertility, alternative sources claim these products can enhance fertility in both men and women. For women, they

---

[67] Aspirin does not prevent pregnancy loss, NIH study finds. (2014, April 1). Retrieved April 3, 2015, from http://www.nih.gov/news/health/apr2014/nichd-01.htm

may help regulate estrogen levels, menstrual cycles, improve egg quality and even help with PMS. In men, they are said to improve sperm quality and output and reduce inflammation of the prostate. For women and couples experiencing miscarriage, bee propolis (the substance used by bees to seal up small openings in their hives) may help with antibodies that attack a developing fetus (similar to an allergic response). Bee propolis may also prevent women's antibodies from attacking sperm. One small study also reported that the use of bee propolis at a dose of 500 mg twice daily resulted in a pregnancy rate of 60% in women with mild endometriosis, as compared to 20% in the placebo group.[68]

Many supplements on the market contain bee pollen, bee propolis and royal jelly. Assuming you do not have an allergy to bees, this may be a great way to supplement your diet. Since brands may differ in concentration and form (i.e. granules or capsules), follow dosing instructions on the product you choose.

---

[68] Ali AFM, Awadallah A. Bee propolis versus placebo in the treatment of infertility, associated with minimal or mild endometriosis: a pilot randomized controlled trial. A modern trend. Fertil Steril . 2003;80 (supp 3):S32.

My Pregnancy Protocol – Part III
Increasing Pelvic Circulation

Water Therapy

I love to take baths, and I know alternating heat and cold to any particular area of your body can increase circulation. I would sit in a tub of ice water for a few minutes, then sit in a hot bathtub for a few minutes alternating back and forth. This helps to increase blood flow to the pelvic region. You may cringe at the thought of sitting in a tub of ice. To help with the discomfort, I got a big plastic storage bin (like the ones you store clothes in), and I would fill it with very cold water in addition to ice cubes. Then, I would place that bin inside the bathtub filled with hot water. You can keep your feet in the hot water while you sit in the ice water and it really helps you withstand the cold. When you've sat in the ice water for a few minutes, you can then easily sit in the tub of hot water right next to the ice tub. Do this as many times a day as you think is realistic (whenever I could, I would take two alternating heat/cold baths per day) but even once a day would be beneficial. I only did this the first half of my cycle because if I did conceive, I did not want the drastic change in temperatures to hurt the fertilized egg or cause me to cramp.

Pelvic Massage

Around the time of ovulation (usually starting about day 11) I would massage my pelvic region especially around my ovaries. I would always massage in a downward or diagonal motion (never up) starting at my ovaries and going down toward my uterus. If you do have a fertilized egg in your tube, you never want it to travel up. During the massage, I would visualize myself assisting the egg out of my ovary into my fallopian tube. I could actually feel when I was ovulating (or near ovulation) because my ovary would swell and be somewhat painful. I previously had my left tube removed, however, we would have intercourse as usual even if I thought I was ovulating on my left (I actually read that in rare cases, the egg can swim to the other side!) Additionally, I had been told by my previous fertility doctor that some women always feel pain on one side even if they're ovulating on the other. So, unless you have an ultrasound, you really can't be sure which side is ovulating.

If you don't know where your ovaries are, they're actually quite low in your pelvis just to the sides of your uterus. They're normally almond shaped, but they can get larger during ovulation. Next time you go to your gynecologist, have them show you exactly where they are if you're unsure. I would continue doing this massage during the week of ovulation and just after so I could not only assist the egg *into* the fallopian tube, but I could also assist it *down* the tube once it was fertilized. This was especially important for me since I had previously had an ectopic (tubal) pregnancy. See also my "Fertility Bodywork" chapter for more in-depth massage techniques.

Evaluate Your Clothing and Shoes

Are your clothes cutting off your pelvic circulation? Refrain from wearing pantyhose or clothes that are too tight in the abdominal region. I remember a few times wearing pantyhose (control top) that were so tight that it would leave a ring around my belly for hours after I took them off. You know that can't be good for your internal organs! Wear breathable fabrics like cotton and try to maintain a comfortable temperature. Tight fitting clothes have been associated with everything from yeast infections to endometriosis. Some theorize that overly tight clothes in the abdominal region might actually drive uterine cells up causing endometriosis. As a matter of fact, populations where women wear loose fitting garments have a much lower incidence of this condition.

Research carried out by Prof. John Dickinson of the Wolfson Institute of Preventive Medicine and published in the British Journal of Obstetrics and Gynecology links tight clothing to endometriosis. The study says tight clothes may provide the force required to drive endometrial cells from the womb to accumulate in the ovaries. They stressed that the garments a woman wears during her menstrual days could be important. "If the garments are so tight-fitting as to produce even a small sustained rise of intra-abdominal solid tissue pressure, retrograde menstruation is likely to occur when the garments are removed and when the salpingo-uterine junction is relaxed between uterine contractions." This is supported by the fact that the condition seems not to exist in countries where loose clothing is the norm. "Almost all women in India wear sarees and have no cosmetic need for constricting garments. Among about 9,000 articles in West African, Central African and East African medical journals, there is only one report of endometriosis from Central Africa."[69]

Moving down to those poor abused feet, I'm a sucker for a good pair of fashionable shoes. Since I'm a petite person, I've always been attracted to high heels. I wore them daily when I worked in the corporate world and I have the bunions to prove it. However, not only do high heels wreak havoc on your feet, they also can hinder your ability

---

[69] Wakhisi, Sylvia. "Why Tight Clothing Exposes You to a Number of Serious Health Risks" Standard Digital. The Nairobian, 29 Mar. 2014. Web. 10 Mar. 2015.http://www.sde.co.ke/thenairobian/article/2000120472/why-tight-clothing-exposes-you-to-a-number-of-serious-health-risks?pageNo=2

to conceive. High heels throw off your center of balance, and to compensate you must tilt the pelvis forward which constricts your pelvic organs.

My Pregnancy Protocol – Part IV
Intercourse

Timing Intercourse

I've read some pretty elaborate methods of predicting ovulation, but I either found them too difficult to follow, or they didn't work. The bottom line is the same as it's been since the beginning of time -- sperm need to be ready and waiting *before* the egg makes its appearance. One study found "among healthy women trying to conceive, nearly all pregnancies can be attributed to intercourse during a six-day period <u>ending</u> on the day of ovulation".[70] I tried to ensure that sperm were available at least 3 days up to and including the day of ovulation (although you can even start 6 days before ovulation as mentioned in the study).

Rather than trying to predict ovulation with predictor kits (which can be quite expensive if you use them regularly), we would have intercourse on days 11, 13, and 15 based on my ovulation history of "day 13". Yes, it is sometimes grueling when neither one wants to have sex (especially on day 15), but for me, it really did work. Having intercourse starting on day 11 and continuing on days 13 and 15 ensured there was always a fresh sperm supply when that egg finally made its way into the fallopian tube. If you have shorter or longer cycles, you will need to revise the dates of intercourse so sperm are available the <u>3 days</u> up to and including your projected ovulation date and possibly a day or two after to account for cycle length variations (that is why we continued having intercourse through day 15). Even though I did not use predictor kits, you may want to

---

[70] Wilcox AJ, Weinberg CR, Baird DD,Timing of sexual intercourse in relation to ovulation. Effects on the probability of conception, survival of the pregnancy, and sex of the baby, N Engl J Med. 1995 Dec 7;333(23):1517-21.

use one for a few months to start just to establish a pattern. If you have very irregular cycles, you may need to continue using them. My cycle did fluctuate slightly from month to month, but having intercourse every other day on cycle days 11-15 was still effective based on my pregnancy history (even with only one fallopian tube). I am somewhat fortunate that I experienced some "mittelschmerz" (ovulation pain), so I usually knew I was "in the ballpark" with my ovulation date, however, unless you have an ultrasound, it's hard to know the exact day of ovulation. When we started fertility treatments (before I tried to conceive naturally), we tried inseminations. The fertility clinic had us use ovulation predictors so we knew which day to go in for the insemination. Since I did have an ultrasound before the procedure to confirm that ovulation was imminent, I can vouch for their accuracy. The other reason I would suggest ovulation predictor kits is because they detect the LH surge *before* ovulation which gives you the chance to have sperm waiting.

I would track my period on my "period calendar" which is just a calendar marking the day I started my period each month so I always knew what day of my cycle I was on (See "Calculating Cycle Days" below).

You can also check the consistency of your vaginal secretions for "fertile mucus". Fertile mucus has the look and feel of egg whites and you tend to have more of it when you're ovulating or just prior to ovulation. Fertile mucus is easier for sperm to swim in and it facilitates the whole process. However, I should mention we stuck with having intercourse on days 11, 13, and 15 whether I had fertile mucus or not. I didn't want to miss any opportunities. Monitoring vaginal secretions, at least for me, was sometimes difficult. As I got older, my vaginal secretions lessened so determining when I was fertile with this method alone was tricky. As a matter of fact, I don't recall having a large amount of fertile mucus the month I conceived my daughter, so I'm glad we didn't rely this method of monitoring my fertility.

I also tried taking my temperature to see when I was ovulating, however, I found my temperature fluctuated so much I really couldn't find a pattern. It was also difficult for me to remember to take my temperature at the same time every day. The other problem is that by the time it goes up, you may have already ovulated. I've talked with a number of doctors about the "temperature" method and they weren't crazy about it. My first fertility doctor came out and said "it doesn't work". One way you could use the temperature method is to establish a pattern of your ovulation cycle day. For that reason, I have included the BBT method at the end of this section.

So, for us, having intercourse three times (every other day) during the week of ovulation was the easiest, least expensive, and most effective (based on results). Having intercourse every other day also will give your partner a chance to replenish his sperm supply. I should mention here that frequency of intercourse is another area where there is conflicting information (some say intercourse every 48 hours, some say daily). For us, being forced into daily intercourse would have added to our stress. You'll have to make your own decision here, but if daily intercourse is too much, every other day should be fine. See also my "Just For Men" chapter for the research on daily intercourse and sperm.

Monitoring ovulation has never been an exact science and recent research has shown it's even less so than previously thought. Many women ovulate or have the potential to ovulate more than once per month, so having intercourse at other times could lead to conception. To further complicate the issue, one study found "in only about 30% of women is the fertile window entirely between days 10 and 17… women can reach their fertile window earlier and others much later. Women should be advised that the timing of their fertile window can be highly unpredictable, even if their cycles are usually regular." [71] This research may support the use of predictor kits due to the extreme variability of ovulation and fertile windows (again, we didn't use predictor kits, but this is probably the only sure method to know if ovulation is about to occur). My husband and I tried to maintain a normal sex life even on weeks I was not ovulating – not only is this good for your relationship, it could lead to pregnancy.

There seems to be differing reports about how long sperm can live, but most sources say up to 5 days inside a woman's body. I can't tell you how many people I've talked to (in the fertile world) who said "I don't know how I got pregnant" because they had intercourse nowhere near their supposed ovulation date. This is why the rhythm method is sometimes very ineffective for couples who are trying to prevent pregnancy.

Sexual Positions For Conception

There isn't solid research that supports any particular position for intercourse to increase your chances of getting pregnant. For us, the missionary position led to all my pregnancies. I found other positions a bit painful probably due to previous surgery and endometriosis. Do not use lubricants. I also kept my feet up in the air after intercourse

---

[71] Wilcox AJ, Dunson D, Baird DD., The timing of the "fertile window" in the menstrual cycle: day specific estimates from a prospective study, BMJ. 2000 Nov 18;321(7271):1259-62.

to help the sperm swim upstream. I would keep my feet up for about 10-15 minutes.

Can You Get Pregnant On Your Period?

This seems to be a very common question. Well…anything is possible, but somewhat unlikely. I suppose if you have very short cycles you could ovulate right after your period ends. Since sperm can live a number of days, you could theoretically get pregnant. I've read that a small percentage of women actually start their fertile window by day four of their menstrual cycle. I'm sure there are those in the fertile world who thought they were safe having intercourse while on their menstrual cycle only to be shocked that they became pregnant.

Calculating Cycle Days

Many women are unclear how to calculate the first day of their menstrual cycle up through the day of ovulation. When I went through fertility treatments, I was given the following guidelines and I've followed them ever since:
1. Day one is the first day of full menstrual flow. If your period starts with spotting, this is not full flow, wait until you see bright red blood.
2. If your period starts late in the day (after 4:00pm) day one should be calculated the following day.
3. Count each day consecutively and start over when your next period begins.

BBT Charting To Establish A Pattern

1. Begin taking your temperature on the first day of your cycle (see above)
2. Take it the same time every day before you get out of bed in the morning and before you eat or drink anything

(you will need to keep a thermometer and chart next to your bed and you may need to set an alarm)
3. Take your temperature orally using a digital thermometer (or check with your local drugstore for a special BBT thermometer)
4. Using a piece of graph paper (or a chart), record your temperature each day with temperature on the left (vertical) with each square representing .1 degree. Put the day on the bottom of the graph (horizontal)
5. After ovulation, your temperature should go up about .1 to .4 degrees. Although this is a small change, it is significant. Your temperature may stay elevated until you get your period again (pregnancy will also keep your temperature elevated.)
6. There might be a very slight dip in temperature immediately preceding ovulation

If you go back and analyze the chart after a month or two, you should see that the "follicular" temperatures (those before ovulation) should be lower and the "luteal" (after ovulation) temperatures should be higher. Again, there are pitfalls to this method because there are things unrelated to ovulation and pregnancy that can affect your BBT. Everything from illness, lack of sleep, too much heat or heated blankets, exhaustion and alcohol can all affect your temperature.

My Pregnancy Protocol – Part V
Other Things To Do Or Avoid

Exercise – How Much is Too Much?

Like many women, I've always had to work at keeping my weight under control. You're always hearing, "diet and exercise", "diet and exercise" and for good reason---it works. But, like many women, I was somewhat of an exercise fanatic. However, it's widely known that overdoing exercise will impair female fertility. One study found, after analyzing women engaging in strenuous exercise, that it affected their ovulatory luteinizing hormone and their menstrual cycles. Six months after the study was over, and the women stopped their rigorous training, their cycles returned to normal.[72] When I went through IVF, my doctor told me I should lay around for 7 days after the embryo transfer and avoid any physical activity. He said their success rates were much higher when women took it easy because implantation was more likely when the body wasn't in motion. Additionally, one study found an increased risk of spontaneous abortion (miscarriage) among the women who reported a high physical strain during the time of implantation of the embryo[73] (see more in my chapter on preventing miscarriage). I got to thinking if my obsession with working out 4-5 times per week was consistent with attaining and maintaining a healthy pregnancy. I had also attended a lecture by an acupuncturist who said most women don't have the "constitution" for heavy exercise.

---

[72] Beverly A. Bullen, Sc.D., Gary S. Skrinar, Ph.D., Inese Z. Beitins, M.D., Gretchen von Mering, B.S., Barry A. Turnbull, M.A., and Janet W. McArthur, M.D., Induction of Menstrual Disorders by Strenuous Exercise in Untrained Women, N Engl J Med 1985; 312:1349-1353May 23, 1985DOI: 10.1056/NEJM198505233122103

[73] Hjollund, Niels Henrik I.; Jensen, Tina Kold; Bonde, Jens Peter E.; More, Spontaneous Abortion and Physical Strain Around Implantation: A Follow-Up Study of First-Pregnancy Planners, Epidemiology. 11(1):18-23, January 2000.

She said sometimes switching to yoga instead of high impact workouts is all some women need to succeed in getting pregnant.

I spent my whole life thinking exercise is a good thing, but now I had to take a hard look at how much was really healthy for my fertility. I decided I would work out only the first half of my cycle up to the day of ovulation. This was a big change for me especially since exercise is something I really enjoy and I was afraid I would gain weight. However, I found if I didn't work out, it was easier to cut down on how much I ate.

My health club offered a number of yoga classes, and I did attend these from time to time. I had to do yoga in moderation because much of the bending was hard on my back (I'm sure it's supposed to help, but for me, it seemed to worsen the back pain I periodically felt). Many people also use yoga as a stress management tool. It helps you focus on your breathing and it's great for stretching tight muscles. Like anything else, you should know your limits whether you're doing yoga or any other type of exercise. I heard an orthopedic surgeon on the radio talking about how he'd seen a number of people actually hurt their joints doing yoga (he recommended pilates). Listen to your body, if it starts to hurt, you know you might need lessen your stretch a bit. I did do some of the yoga poses recommended in my "Fertility Bodywork" chapter on my own outside of a yoga class.

If you are someone who has not exercised in the past, start taking walks (but only in the first half of your cycle). You want your body to be healthy, but now is not the time to become an olympic athlete.

Weight and Fertility

There is evidence that optimum fertility occurs when you're not too thin or too heavy. A study done on weight and conception reported: "obesity has been observed to impair both natural and assisted conception. The exact pathophysiological mechanism through which obesity exerts its detrimental effect remains uncertain. It is likely that obesity exerts its effect upon conception and implantation through a cumulative impairment of several processes. Obesity affects ovulation, oocyte maturation, endometrial development, uterine receptivity, implantation and miscarriage."[74] I also address weight in my chapter on preventing miscarriage.

Try to maintain a healthy weight for your body type. If you're overweight, adding the fruits and vegetables and walking should help you reduce your weight in a slow and healthy fashion. If you're too thin, try cutting down on exercise but maintain a healthy diet. Being too thin or too heavy definitely has an effect on hormones. Women and girls who work out excessively or women who get too thin stop getting their periods. It's also believed that women who are overweight store extra estrogen in their fat cells. This may be why young girls who are overweight tend to get their periods earlier than average. Excess estrogen can lead to many conditions which cause or contribute to infertility.

Since most Americans have a tendency to be overweight, let me say here that obesity isn't just linked to infertility, it has also been linked to premature births, and even birth

---

[74] Christopher J Brewer and Adam H Balen, Focus on Obesity: The adverse effects of obesity on conception and implantation, Reproduction 140 (3) 347-364, doi: 10.1530/REP-09-0568 First published online 15 April 2010

defects.[75] You should address your weight issues *before* you try to conceive because you don't want to be dieting when pregnant. There also seems to be evidence that conception is less likely to occur when body weight is declining.

Here is a chart which should help you evaluate whether or not your weight is in the normal range by calculating your body mass index or BMI:

1. Multiply your weight in pounds by 703 and divide that number by your height in inches
2. Divide the result of #1 again by your height in inches

A score below 18.5 indicates being underweight.
Between 18.5 and 24.9 means a healthy body weight.
Between 25 and 29.9 means you are overweight.
Between 30 and 39.9 indicates obesity
A score of 40 or higher indicates morbid obesity

Sunlight

Getting enough sunlight can be a critical piece of maximizing your fertility. The reason is sunlight can promote ovulation. Supposedly, one reason why many people who go on vacation get pregnant is they're finally outdoors long enough to get some sunlight. Now, I'm not talking about staying outside all day, just maybe one hour per day. You really do feel better when you get outside for a while – especially if you've been a workaholic, you may have forgotten what it's like to soak in the fresh air. I always visualized the sun ripening my eggs. If you spend most of your day cooped up in an office, spend your lunch

---

[75] Waller DK, Shaw GM, Rasmussen SA, Hobbs CA, Canfield MA, Siega-Riz AM, Gallaway MS, Correa A. Prepregnancy obesity as a risk factor for structural birth defects. Archives of Pediatrics & Adolescent Medicine. 2007; 161(8):745-750.

hour outside or take a walk on your breaks. After I quit my job I would designate an hour every morning as my outdoor time. Fortunately, I live in an area where the sun shines daily, but if you don't, you may have to get out there when the opportunity arises. For the maximum effect, make sure the sunlight actually hits your eyes (again, only about an hour per day). The full spectrum light provided from the sun is important to maintain normal circadian rhythms and to re-set your body clock. Sunlight helps regulate your sleep-wake cycle which will help with melatonin production discussed in the next section. If weather permits, let the sun hit your arms and legs for the first 20 minutes to absorb vitamin D.

Also of note is the findings of one study on light and women's ovulation which reported: "morning exposure to bright light in the follicular phase of the menstrual cycle stimulates the secretion of hypophyseal reproductive hormones, promotes ovary follicle growth, and increases ovulation rates in women with slightly lengthened menstrual cycles. This might be a promising method to overcome infertility."[76] Although this study was done with artificial light, it seems that light has a relationship to balancing reproductive hormones.

Earthing

There is a practice called "earthing" which is simply walking barefoot on grass, soil, sand and so on. Whenever possible get outside (perhaps while on a walk to get your sunlight) and remove your shoes on non-paved or non-concrete earth surfaces. Better yet, sit directly on the grass while you eat your lunch. This is thought to draw electrons

---

[76] Danilenko, K. V., & Samoilova, E. A. (2007). Stimulatory Effect of Morning Bright Light on Reproductive Hormones and Ovulation: Results of a Controlled Crossover Trial. PLoS Clinical Trials, 2(2), e7. doi:10.1371/journal.pctr.0020007

from the earth which has been associated with a number of health benefits including stress reduction and regulating our biological clocks and rhythms. One study found, "The research done to date supports the concept that grounding or earthing the human body may be an essential element in the health equation."[77]

Sleep

Another extremely important factor in increasing your overall health and fertility is getting an adequate amount of sleep. It was found in one study that women who got adequate sleep had reproductive hormones that were 20% higher than those who did not. [78]

Melatonin is a hormone which is stimulated by darkness and regulates sleep. A lack of Melatonin may have an adverse effect on female reproductive hormones. Get some blackout shades/curtains (or cut some cardboard to fit the shape of your windows) so you can keep your room as dark as possible in the morning. This will help stimulate Melatonin production. I found I was able to sleep much longer in the morning after installing black out curtains.

Also of note, it was found that women who go bed by 10:00pm have a lower risk of breast cancer. It is thought that their melatonin levels decreased their estrogen production thereby decreasing their risk for hormone related cancers. Melatonin is also a powerful antioxidant and can prevent cell damage. Even though regulating your

---

[77] Chevalier, G., Sinatra, S. T., Oschman, J. L., Sokal, K., & Sokal, P. (2012). Earthing: Health Implications of Reconnecting the Human Body to the Earth's Surface Electrons. Journal of Environmental and Public Health, 2012, 291541. doi:10.1155/2012/291541

[78] Sandrine Touzet, Muriel Rabilloud, Hans Boehringer, Enriqueta Barranco, René Ecochard, Relationship between sleep and secretion of gonadotropin and ovarian hormones in women with normal cycles, Fertility and Sterility, Volume 77, Issue 4, April 2002, Pages 738-744

melatonin levels naturally is a good thing, larger doses of melatonin can suppress ovulation[79], so taking supplements is probably not a good idea.

Once I quit my job, I was able to easily get 9 hours of sleep every night. When I was working, I would normally go to bed around 11:00pm and get up at 6:00am. Many times I wouldn't get a good night's sleep because I was tossing and turning and worrying about some crisis at work. For me, getting a good night's sleep is one of the most luxurious and satisfying experiences I can think of. I also found when I was able to get sound sleep I actually would dream about the baby who was going to come into my life. I would frequently dream I was pregnant or I would dream about having a baby/child. You actually have power over what you dream at night. Before you go to sleep, tell yourself what you would like to dream about. You'll be surprised, it really does work!

Blood Pressure

I have a chapter devoted to evaluating your stress level and methods of stress reduction, so I won't address that here. However, I do want to mention that you should keep an eye on your blood pressure. Is your blood pressure *below* 120/80? If not, this may be an indicator your stress level is too high (although many people have high blood pressure whether under stress or not). I do recall having intermittent high blood pressure readings when I would take time out of my work day for doctor appointments. After I quit my job, my blood pressure readings were always normal.

High blood pressure is something that can really get out of control during pregnancy, so you want to address it now.

---

[79] The Miracle of Melatonin? (1995, October 1). Retrieved April 3, 2015, from http://acsh.org/1995/10/the-miracle-of-melatonin/

In terms of *getting* pregnant, there is evidence high blood pressure can negatively affect fertility in both men and women. There may even be an association between hypertension and uterine fibroids because the increased pressure may cause uterine muscle injury[80]. If you have high blood pressure, this is really something you should monitor with your physician. Left unchecked, it can be very serious and even life threatening over time. I actually knew a woman who went through IVF, gave birth to twins, and died from a stroke postpartum because her blood pressure was so high. I don't say this to scare you, but it emphasizes the importance of staying on top of it.

A word of warning: there is a classification of antihypertensive medications called ACE inhibitors which have been linked to birth defects when women used them early in pregnancy.[81] If you do need to go on medication for hypertension, be sure to bring this up with your doctor. I certainly don't want to discourage you from taking high blood pressure medication if you need it, but you should be aware of this risk with ACE inhibitors. There are different types of antihypertensive medications which are probably safer for women who are trying to conceive.

Having said that, there is much you can do to control your blood pressure naturally. Everything in my pregnancy protocol is great for overall health, weight and blood pressure. But some people have hypertension unrelated to their lifestyle. It's probably a good idea to check your blood pressure frequently since one reading may not give a complete picture. Most drugstores, discounts stores, and

---

[80] Brookes, L. (n.d.). Hypertension Associated With Presence of Fibroids in Premenopausal Women. Retrieved April 1, 2015, from http://www.medscape.org/viewarticle/502862_6
[81] Cooper WO, Hernandez-Diaz S, Arbogast PG, Dudley JA, Dyer S, Gideon PS, et al. Major congenital malformations after first-trimester exposure to ACE inhibitors. N Engl J Med. 2006;354:2443–51.

grocery stores now have machines that will take your blood pressure for free. When I was trying to conceive and during my entire pregnancy, I would check my blood pressure at least once per week on these machines. I've heard some doctors say that these machines may not be accurate, so just to be sure, I would check it at a different store every week. I would usually get consistent readings, so I knew my blood pressure was in the normal range. The other nice thing about checking your blood pressure on a machine is that you won't suffer from what they call "white coat syndrome". This is when your blood pressure goes up just from the stress of having a doctor or other healthcare person check it. There is some research that people with white coat syndrome may be more prone to having high blood pressure because the way they react to this type of stress may indicate a similar reaction to other stressful situations. But in any event, at least you will know what your blood pressure is in a normal situation.

Prolactin and Fertility

Prolactin is a hormone which is best known for being responsible for milk production in lactating mothers. However, it is a hormone that is present in both men and women. When prolactin is elevated, it affects ovulation and menstrual cycles. This is why you've probably heard that breastfeeding women won't get pregnant (although this is not always true, many lactating women do get pregnant). Prolactin can have an effect on other hormones involved with the reproductive system. If you are trying to conceive, and you have elevated prolactin (unrelated to pregnancy), this could be problematic. One study found: "elevated prolactin may impact reproduction through inhibitory effects on hypothalamic gonadotropin-releasing hormone (GnRH) neurons and/or on the pituitary gland to reduce secretion of the gonadotropins luteinizing hormone (LH) and follicle-stimulating hormone (FSH), resulting in a reduction in both amplitude and frequency of LH pulses."[82]

Hyperprolactinemia, can also cause discharge from the breasts. Men may also experience infertility as a result of elevated prolactin. It can lead to problems with sperm production and erectile dysfunction. If you have symptoms of hyperprolactinemia, of course, you should talk with your doctor because there are certain tumors that can cause this condition and it can be caused or made worse from some prescription medications. Women with thyroid disorders or PCOS may also be at higher risk for elevated prolactin. However, in addition to medical therapy, there are natural ways to help with this condition. They include:

1. Eating foods high in vitamin B6 - this includes chicken, salmon, potatoes, spinach
2. Increasing intake of zinc - eat foods like beans which are natural sources of zinc
3. Vitex or Chasteberry
4. Vitamin E (this may work even better if combined with vitamin B6 as mentioned above)
5. Eating foods high in phytoestrogens - The theory here is that higher estrogen levels will suppress prolactin. As explained earlier, phytoestrogens are plant based estrogens which are weaker than the ones produced by your body, but they are considered safer than synthetic estrogens. As mentioned in my fertility diet, foods high in phytoestrogens include: soy, flax seeds, many nuts like walnuts, almonds, pistachios, hazelnuts, many legumes, and other foods like broccoli, and cabbage.

---

[82] Kaiser, U. B. (2012). Hyperprolactinemia and infertility: new insights. The Journal of Clinical Investigation, 122(10), 3467–3468. doi:10.1172/JCI64455

Thyroid and Fertility

A number of lifestyle factors can influence how the thyroid functions. For instance, poor nutrition, high levels of stress, infections, exposure to environmental radiation, toxins and even fluoride can throw the thyroid out of whack. You may also have a genetic predisposition to thyroid irregularities. According to one study, "abnormalities in thyroid function, including hyperthyroidism and hypothyroidism, can have an adverse effect on reproductive health and result in reduced rates of conception, increased early pregnancy loss, and adverse pregnancy and neonatal outcomes."[83]

If the thyroid is underperforming (hypothyroidism), a woman may have the following problems:
- lack of ovulation
- short menstrual cycles
- hormone regulation problems like high prolactin, estrogen dominance, low progesterone

Hyperthyroidism (over-production) is less common and may require medication or possibly surgery. If it is left untreated and a woman becomes pregnant, it could lead to a number of pregnancy complications or miscarriage. If the thyroid is overproducing, you may be experiencing the following:
- feeling irritable or nervous
- weight loss
- sweating
- rapid heartbeat

Based on my research, if you are experiencing the more common "hypothyroidism" there are ways you can help the condition it naturally. These include:

---

[83] Jefferys A, Vanderpump M, Yasmin E. Thyroid dysfunction and reproductive health. The Obstetrician & Gynaecologist 2015;17:39–45.

- Yoga poses that increase circulation to the area around the thyroid. The "Shoulder stand" is one example (this is a pose where you are laying on your back with your legs and lower back raised with most of your weight in the shoulder area and hands supporting your lower back).
- General Exercise: This helps to increase metabolism and counteract weight gain.
- Sunlight and/or 2000iu of Vitamin D
- Fish Oils (about 2 grams per day)
- Make sure you are getting enough iodine (iodized salt and seaweed may be sources)
- Selenium
- Herbs such as black cohosh, hypericum and cayenne
- Drink plenty of water
- Avoid soy: As I mentioned in my fertility food section, critics of soy are concerned with its goitrogenic activity which can lead to thyroid disruptions. Again, I did consume soy when I was trying to conceive and it is found as part of my fertility diet, but I had never been diagnosed with a thyroid disorder or an iodine deficiency.

Of course, these natural methods are not a substitute for medical advice and treatment and you should have your thyroid levels checked and follow the advice of your doctor.

Gum Disease

Women who are trying to conceive should maintain their oral health. According to one study, "the presence of periodontal disease is a modifiable risk factor, which can increase a woman's time to conception."[84]

Things to Avoid

- Genetically Modified Foods: GMO stands for genetically modified organisms and they are being produced like never before and they are already in our food supply. There are some scary statistics out there, here are a few reported by the Institute for Responsible Technology:
Hamsters Fed GMOS became sterile by the third generation
More than half of baby rats died after their mothers ate GMO's (and they were smaller)
Female rats who ate GMO's had changes in their reproductive system, including ovaries and uterus
Male rats had changes in testicles and sperm development[85]
Although these are animal studies, it may be worth buying organic non-GMO food from your local health food store.

- Do not consume foods with 'trans fats'. Trans fats are extremely harmful substances which not only clog your arteries, but they can affect fertility by interfering with hormone production (they may also be associated with miscarriage). Trans fats are most commonly found in convenience foods like cookies, crackers, and many packaged dry goods and frozen dinners. Read the labels and don't buy anything that has "partially hydrogenated vegetable oil". Trans fats are made from

---

[84] European Society of Human Reproduction and Embryology (ESHRE). "Gum disease can increase the time it takes to become pregnant." ScienceDaily. ScienceDaily, 1 August 2011. <www.sciencedaily.com/releases/2011/07/110705071548.htm>
[85] Health Risks Of GMO's. (n.d.). Retrieved April 3, 2015, from http://www.responsibletechnology.org/health-risks

vegetable oils through a process called hydrogenation, which involves mixing liquid oils with hydrogen atoms to make them solid and prevent them going bad. Trans fats interfere with the formation of the good prostaglandins. When I started diligently reading labels, I was appalled at how contaminated our food supply is! For cooking and baking, experts on food and nutrition are now saying that you're better off using butter rather than margarine since margarine is made from partially hydrogenated vegetable oil. The best thing to do, in my opinion, is to use olive oil, coconut oil, or some of the new "buttery spreads" that say "no trans fats or hydrogenated oils" (these are made from vegetable oils). If you use vegetable oils, refrigerate them to keep them from going rancid. The FDA has started requiring manufacturers of food products to place clearly on their labels the amount of trans fats their product contains. Many food manufacturers have voluntarily taken trans fats out of their foods and have actually started fortifying them with the healthy Omega-3 fats.

- Do not consume soft drinks because of an ingredient called "sodium benzoate". When this is combined with vitamin C which is also in many soft drinks, it forms something called benzene. Benzene can cause cell death. If you enjoy carbonated beverages, try seltzer water. I frequently mix natural seltzer water with my cold tea for a healthy carbonated drink.

- Do not consume the artificial sweetener "aspartame". There is conflicting information on the safety of using aspartame before and during pregnancy, however you should know that some sources have linked aspartame to infertility, birth defects and even some cancers. I'm not a researcher, so I can't tell you who is right, but just to be on the safe side, I cut aspartame out of my diet when I was trying to conceive. Stevia may be a safer alternative.

- Do not use sunscreens which have the following ingredients: octinoxate, oxybenzone, PABA or padimate O. These ingredients may mimic estrogen. Try to stick with zinc oxide and titanium dioxide.

- Do not consume the flavor enhancer, MSG (Monosodium Glutamate). It is found in many packaged products like soups, flavored chips and seasoning packets.

- Do not use scented tampons, or vaginal sprays. These products can cause irritation which may lead to infections. Douching has also been studied and found to reduce fertility.[86]

- Do not expose yourself to toxic substances or radiation – stay away from pesticides, herbicides (these are xenoestrogens), solvents, and cleaning products that have warning labels. For the most part, I've made the transition to cleaning with natural substances like water, vinegar and baking soda. This will be another bonus when you have a toddler running around getting into things – what could be better than edible cleaning products? If you must come in contact with substances you are unsure of, use a mask and gloves. If you have a job where you're exposed to any sort of radiation, you really need to evaluate how safe it is to continue working – especially when you get pregnant, you don't

---

[86] D D Baird, C R Weinberg, L F Voigt, and J R Daling, Vaginal douching and reduced fertility, Am J Public Health. 1996 June; 86(6): 844–850.

want your baby exposed. I knew a fertility doctor who wouldn't let his clients take airplane flights because of the amount of radiation they were exposed to. Based on my reading, an occasional short flight isn't going to expose you to dangerous amounts of radiation, but if you travel frequently, that may be another story. I rarely traveled when I was trying to get pregnant (maybe once a year) so this wasn't an issue for me, but if I was anywhere near ovulation, I would avoid getting mammograms, dental x-rays, etc.

- Do not sleep on heated waterbeds or electric blankets or unplug them while you're in bed. I had a waterbed during the time I was trying to conceive and during my pregnancy. The waterbed was wonderful when I was pregnant because it had a lot of "give" which is much more comfortable when your belly is large. But I *always* unplugged it before I got in it. During the summer months, I kept it unplugged all the time.

- Do not use products with "parabens". Look at the labels of your shampoo, lotion, and other cosmetics. If they have methylparaben, propylparaben, butylparaben or any other ingredient that ends in "paraben", do not use them. I was able to find plenty of over the counter brands that do not contain these ingredients. These parabens are xenoestrogens which may throw your hormones out of balance. Another scary statistic is that studies have shown that parabens can accumulate in the body and have been found in breast tissue and breast tumors (methylparaben was present at the highest level).[87] Now that I have my daughter, I continue to

---

87 Darbre, P. D., Aljarrah, A., Miller, W. R., Coldham, N. G., Sauer, M. J. and Pope, G. S. (2004), Concentrations of parabens in human breast tumours. J. Appl. Toxicol., 24: 5–13. doi: 10.1002/jat.958

My Specific Pregnancy Protocol

watch out for these ingredients which are even in many baby and children's products.

- Do not heat food or water in plastic containers. The plastic may diffuse into the food or water and act as xenoestrogens which again, can throw your hormones out of balance. Also watch out for canned foods (the cans are lined with plastic) and even plastic silverware. Bisphenol A (found in some plastics) may be linked to miscarriage and birth defects. It may be impossible to avoid it completely, but try to eliminate your exposure as much as possible.

- Do not re-use plastic bottles to drink water or other beverages for the same reason listed above. Also, do not freeze water in plastic bottles. If you want to be environmentally friendly by reusing drinking bottles, go out and buy a beverage in a glass bottle (with a screw on cap) then wash and reuse.

- Do not use commercial laundry detergent. Much of it does not rinse out of your clothes and rubs off on your skin acting as a xenoestrogen. Try using things like Borax or organic detergent from your health food store. If you do you use commercial laundry detergent, try using less than the recommended amount (try pre-treating tough stains which will help you use less.) Run your clothes through two rinse cycles and avoid fabric softeners and dryer sheets. If you need a fabric softener, try baking soda.

- Do not drink alcohol – at least in the second half of your menstrual cycle (past day 14). You don't want to find out you're pregnant after you "tied one on"! Personally, I rarely drank alcohol while I was trying to conceive. If I was going to have alcohol, I would only have a glass of wine when I was on my period (usually with dinner).

- Let's not forget the obvious…do not smoke! Of course you already know this one but I feel obligated to mention it can be a major source of infertility. Also, smoking can actually damage egg quality and it can affect uterine receptivity to a fertilized egg.

- Do not use "antibacterial" soaps. The ingredient "triclosan" hinders an enzyme linked to the metabolism of estrogen.[88] Most people really don't need "antibacterial" soaps anyway. Regular soap usually does the trick. If you must use hand sanitizers, make sure they are triclosan free. This ingredient is also in some toothpastes.

---

[88] Antibacterial agent could cause pregnancy problems. (2010, November 4). Retrieved from http://news.ufl.edu/archive/2010/11/antibacterial-agent-could-cause-pregnancy-problems.html

Chapter 4
Fertility Bodywork

Pelvic Massage and Increasing Pelvic circulation

There are a number of techniques you can perform on yourself which can enhance pelvic circulation and even break up small blockages. There are also some yoga poses and routines you can follow to improve your fertility. You should run through these practices daily (unless otherwise specified). My video, "Fertility Bodywork" demonstrates these techniques as well.

Yoga Poses:

1. The Bridge Pose - the bridge stimulates abdominal organs and can relieve menstrual discomfort if done regularly. It calms the brain and can help with stress. Start by lying with your back on the floor. Bend your knees, put your feet flat on the floor as close to your buttocks as possible. While tucking your tailbone under, bring your buttocks and back up until you form a bridge and bring your hands together clasped underneath you. Hold this pose for 30 seconds to one minute.

2. The Cobbler's Pose - this pose also stimulates abdominal organs, ovaries and is thought to be a natural remedy for infertility. Sit on the floor, bend your knees and let them lay out to the side while pressing down toward the floor with your thighs. Bring your feet together and hold the toes

or ankles with your hands. You may stay in this pose for 1-5 minutes.

3. The Lotus pose - this pose stimulates the pelvis, spine, abdomen and bladder. It can help ease the pain of childbirth if done throughout pregnancy. This pose starts by sitting cross legged on the floor. Slowly bring one foot on top of your thigh then the other foot on top of the other thigh. If this is painful, you may stay seated cross legged without the feet on the thighs. Bring your thumb and middle fingers together and rest on your knees. You may stay in this pose for as long as it is comfortable or for about 5 minutes.

4. The Reclining Hero pose - this pose probably needs to be done with support (a bolster pillow can be used along the length of your back). The reclining hero pose helps to open up and stretch the abdomen and it can ease menstrual pain. This pose begins by kneeling then sitting down between your feet then slowly reclining down until you are laying on the floor. You may need to bring your knees up a little but keep your thighs parallel. Keep your pelvis tucked under and lengthen your back. You may lay your arms out diagonally away from your body on the floor. This is an intermediate pose and you may need additional support with a second pillow on your back until you become more experienced. You may stay in this pose 30 seconds to one minute and longer as you get more experienced.

5. Legs up the wall pose - Find a blank wall in your home and lay down with your buttocks up against the wall. Use a rolled up blanket or bolster pillow to support your lower back. Raise your legs so they are up against the wall. They do not have to be completely straight. Spread your shoulder blades out and lay the hands to the sides and above your head. You may stay in this pose for 5-15 minutes. This pose is good for ovarian problems in women and semen or

testicular problems in men. It increases pelvic circulation and it can help with adrenal and thyroid function. After intercourse, it can help with deeper penetration of semen. Do not do this pose during menstruation as you do not want backflow, however if it is done other times during the month, it can help decrease menstrual pain when you are on your cycle.

Pelvic Massage Techniques

My Fertility Bodywork Video demonstrates these techniques, but here are some pelvic massages you can perform on yourself. It is not recommended to do any of these techniques if there is any possibility that you may already be pregnant. You should also refrain from these techniques if you are on your menstrual cycle:

1. Uterine Lift

Many women carry their uterus too low because of past sports and exercise, trauma and heavy lifting. The uterine lift can put the uterus back into its proper position which will help with the proper flow of blood, lymphatic fluids and nerve impulses. First, find your uterus by making a triangle with your thumbs and forefingers with the thumbs at the navel. The uterus should be at the tips of the forefingers. Move down to the bottom of the uterus which should be just above the pubic bone. Push down and try to scoop the uterus up with your fingers toward your navel. Hold for about 30 seconds and release.

2. Uterine Massage

First, find your uterus with the triangle mentioned above with your thumbs and forefingers. Start the massage with an up and down motion along the uterus. Then, using moderate pressure, massage the uterus along an imaginary circle on the outside of the uterus and then an inner circle on the uterus. The massage will consist of small circular motions with your index and middle fingers. To finish, roll over on your stomach and pat your lower back.

3. Femoral Massage

This massage temporarily saturates the pelvic vessels with blood by putting pressure on the femoral artery and releasing. As with all of these techniques, do not perform if you may be pregnant or on your menstrual cycle. Additionally, the femoral massage should not be done if you have heart disease, high blood pressure, thrombosis, varicose veins, phlebitis, history of aneurysm, stroke or other circulatory problems.

Locate the femoral artery in your groin area just under the crease between your thigh and your lower abdomen. You usually know when you have found it because you will feel a strong pulsing sensation. Press down firmly until the pulsing stops. Hold the pressure for about 30 seconds before releasing. When you release the pressure, you should feel a very warm sensation. Repeat this two more times. The entire sequence can be done twice per day on both sides.

4. Fallopian Tube Massage

The fallopian tube massage can help to reduce and loosen blockages and adhesions in the area. It should not be done in the second half of your cycle or during menstruation. I should mention that immediately after ovulation, I did lightly massage my one remaining fallopian tube in a downward motion in hopes that if there was a fertilized egg, it would keep moving downward.

Find your uterus with the triangle and go outward about two inches. Massage in a circular motion back and forth within the two inches toward your uterus. Do this massage for 5-15 minutes every day on both sides. End by pressing the area with the heel of your hand.

5. Ovarian Massage

This massage helps relieve tension and congestion in the ovaries. If you have ovarian cysts, this may be painful and you should lighten the pressure. Start by going out three inches from your navel and down about four inches to find your ovaries. Massage with your index and middle fingers with moderate pressure in a circular motion. Complete about 30 circles on each side and end by pressing the area with the heel of your hand.

My Fertility Bodywork video also covers acupressure and reflexology which you may perform on yourself. They are not covered here because they are best learned through visual demonstration.

Castor Oil Packs

When I was trying to conceive, I had heard of pelvic massage, but I did not know about the benefits of castor oil and castor oil packs. I knew about taking castor oil internally and the benefits of the "good fats", but using it externally was new to me. Castor oil is probably something your grandmother used to treat all sorts of problems because it can be used as a laxative, antimicrobial and as a way to stimulate your immune system. But what about its external uses? When castor oil is applied to the skin, it is absorbed and is thought to increase lymphocytes. These lymphocytes aide the removal of toxins from your body. Edgar Cayce was one of the pioneers in the use of external castor oil and recommended the use of castor oil packs. Castor oil packs, when used externally on your abdomen, can also help with pelvic circulation. You can buy these pre-made, but if you have a few minutes, you can easily make them yourself. Here are instructions:

1. Heat ⅓ cup organic castor oil in a heat-safe bowl (it is not recommended to microwave the castor oil, heat the oil with a "double boiler"). Be sure to use moderate heat as you don't want to burn your skin.
2. Cut a piece of flannel large enough to cover your abdomen (perhaps from an old blanket which has been washed with hypoallergenic detergent).
3. After the castor oil is heated, saturate the flannel completely, but make sure it is not dripping.
4. Get an old fashioned water bottle and fill with moderately hot water.
5. Lay on an old blanket or towel so you don't get oil on your furniture.
6. Cover your abdomen with the oil saturated flannel.
7. Put a piece of plastic over the flannel (so you don't get oil on your clothes or the hot water bottle).
8. Put the hot water bottle on top of the plastic.
9. Lay here for 30-40 minutes.

It is recommended to use castor oil packs 4 days on, 3 days off per week for 4-6 weeks. You should avoid using them during your menstrual cycle or if you think you may be pregnant so use the first half of your cycle.

Chapter 5
Alternative Techniques

Emotional Freedom Technique

The Emotional Freedom Technique is sometimes called "emotional acupuncture" without needles. It is also called "tapping" because it involves tapping acupuncture points along the energy meridians. It helps to release blockages created with emotional stress. Going through infertility can be a source of these blockages and those very blockages can prevent your pregnancy. EFT is something you can perform on yourself and it is thought to have very high success rates.

So how do you perform EFT?

First of all, you need a "set up phrase". This is related to the part of your life which is causing stress and emotional blockages. If you are experiencing infertility, your set up phrase might be:

"Even though I am experiencing infertility, I deeply and completely accept myself...I am ready to have a child now".

One thing I had to get used to with EFT is that it recommends focusing on the issue that is giving you trouble. Much of what I had learned previously taught the power of positive thinking and focusing on success, not the cause of failure. However, EFT differs in this respect. It focuses on the issue causing the disruption to stimulate the energy pathways to balance it out.

Now you are ready for the tapping phase. You are going to lightly tap the following areas while repeating your set-up phrase:

- Karate Chop Point (on the side of your hand between the bottom of your small finger and the bottom of your palm).
- Top of the Head (TOH) - This point will be the center of your head.
- Beginning of the Eyebrow (EB) to the side and above the nose.
- Side of the Eye (SE) This will be on the outside corner of the eye.
- Under the Eye (UE) This will be the center of the underside of the eye.
- Under the Nose (UN) This will be directly under the center of the nose.
- Chin Point (CH) This will be the center of your chin.
- Beginning of the Collarbone (CB) This is to the right (or left) of the area where a man's tie would knot.
- Under the Arm (UA) This is centered about 4" below the armpit where your bra would go around from your front to your back.

It doesn't matter which side of your body you tap (right or left is fine). If you are right handed, it may be easier to tap with your right hand on the left side of your body. You will tap each of the points listed above about 7 times while repeating the set up phrase. Tap each point with your index and middle finger firmly but not so hard as to cause pain. You will go through all of the points in order while repeating your phrase. The next step is to go through all the points again using a reminder phrase. This is basically the same as a set-up phrase, but you can shorten it to "remind" yourself which issue you are clearing from your body. So instead of saying "Even though I am experiencing infertility, I deeply and completely accept myself...I am ready to have a child now", you might just say "I am experiencing infertility". If you choose to use the entire set up phrase in the second round, that's fine too. EFT can be done right before your visualization and meditation discussed in the next chapter.

Feng Shui for Fertility

Feng shui was originally developed in China and it is considered both an art and a science. If you are wondering exactly what feng shui means, the word "feng" means wind, and the word "shui" means water. It is thought that our spaces are filled with energy or "chi". One goal is to make sure that your living area has positive energy flow. So how can feng shui help with fertility and getting pregnant? Your environment can help create positive baby "chi". Here are some of the design principles of feng shui for fertility:

- Clear out clutter in your home that might be blocking energy flow. This also makes room for a baby in your life.
- Remove ceiling fans and large light fixtures over your bed - this is thought to empty the energy around the solar plexus which might prevent a pregnancy from implanting or growing.
- Remove mirrors from your bedroom and keep mirrors away from your front door. Mirrors are thought to push away energy.
- Keep electronic devices away from your bed.

- Remove everything from under your bed and do not store household items or clothing under your bed.
- Once you have removed items and clutter from under your bed, place a bowl of uncooked rice underneath it. This is thought to improve the fertility of those sleeping in the bed above. Before the dangers to birds were known, uncooked white rice was thrown at weddings to wish children upon the newlyweds.
- Refrain from cleaning or disturbing the space underneath the bed from this point forward. It is thought that your future child's soul may visit and hide under the bed.
- Place a fertility symbol in your bedroom: elephants (with their trunk facing down) symbolize fertility. Place this in the west or northwest direction.
- Avoid the color red in your bedroom as it is too hot and is thought to drain the baby energy. Try to incorporate calming and gender-neutral colors like white, tan, ivory and gold.
- Add a water feature to your house and bedroom like a small fountain.
- Place a small dragon symbol or charm near your bed to conjure up yang energy to help you conceive.
- Make sure there is nothing but open space in your entry area outside your front door. If you have a busy street, trees or other obstructions outside your front door, try placing wind chimes on either side of the front door to counteract the obstruction.
- Put a bowl of pomegranates (which symbolize fertility) in your bedroom, but keep them fresh. You could also hang a picture of a pair of pomegranates.
- Hang pictures of babies or children in your bedroom, or hang your vision board (discussed next chapter) on one of your walls.
- Consider using green sheets (which are thought to enhance fertility) on your bed and paint the wall behind

the bed yellow or put a large yellow wall hanging behind the bed (the color of children).
- If you have children or babies in your home as guests, allow them to sit or play on your bed. This is supposed to attract babies and children to you.
- Eliminate "poison arrows" near your front door and in your bedroom. These are sharp angular objects which create sharp corners pointing at you. You can cover them up with plants, but don't use plants that have sharp leaves creating more arrows.
- Add a figure or statue of Buddha with children in the West area of your bedroom. Do not place this figure on the floor.
- Place a hollow piece of bamboo in the west area of the bedroom. This symbolizes growth, flexibility and freedom.

Chapter 6
Visualization, Meditation and Changing Your Pregnancy Mindset for Conception

If you've been on the career track most of your life, you probably haven't had time to sit and meditate. Initially, for me, meditation brought to mind images of incense burning, warped string instruments, and frizzy headed throwbacks from the sixties humming and sitting cross legged on the floor. It really doesn't have to be like that. Meditation can be done anywhere and anytime when you can have uninterrupted quiet for at least 15 minutes. I would frequently meditate in the bathtub. First of all, it's uninterrupted time, second, it's probably one of the few times all your muscles are relaxed.

Visualization and Meditation

I would follow a routine of first visualizing, then doing meditation. What's the difference? Visualization is when you actually daydream about what you want. I would visualize my baby. I would see pictures in my mind of me holding my baby, rocking her to sleep, feeding her, or just playing and laughing with her (somehow I guess I knew I was going to have a girl). I would look around at other babies and imagine how my baby might look. I would see a cute outfit and think *my baby is going to look great in that*! I would see someone with their baby in a front pack and I would imagine myself with my baby sleeping next to my chest. I would see babies in restaurants and I would see myself feeding my baby.

Meditation, on the other hand, is when you think of absolutely nothing. You train your mind to be blank. It is during this quieting of the mind you connect to the power of the universe where anything is possible. It takes practice and discipline to turn off the "chatter" in your mind. I found it helpful to focus on the space between my upper and lower eyelids. When my eyes were closed, I could see a faint line of light where my eyelids met. I would always bring myself back to this line of light whenever my mind started drifting off. Meditation is also a great stress management tool. I would always feel very relaxed (but not sleepy) after I meditated. It is such a relief to think of nothing – even if it's only for 15 minutes at a time. I found it helpful to first visualize, then meditate. That way, you tell the universe what you want (visualization), then you connect yourself to the universal power to get it (meditation). I did find it helpful to burn a candle during this process. There's something about a flame flickering that really brings you back to nature and connects you to a higher power.

I found myself using any downtime for visualization (even if I couldn't actually meditate). If I had to wait somewhere in line, I would sit and daydream about my baby. Once, I accidentally locked myself out of the house without my phone, so I used this time for visualization and meditation until my husband got home (even though I was sitting on my front porch!) I *can* get pregnant, I would continually tell myself. Look at all of the miraculous things my body can do! It can breathe on its own, it can think on its own, it can take food, digest it, convert it to energy – none of these things are easy! If my body can do all of these things, it can make a healthy, happy baby!

Since I also had a problem with miscarriage. I would visualize a little angel with wings fluttering inside of me guiding the fertilized egg down my fallopian tube and into my uterus. I would visualize the egg attaching high in my uterus and the angel would make sure it was a firm and secure attachment. I would visualize the angel taking care of my baby all throughout my successful pregnancy. I also would picture myself lying down with a beam of light shining down from the heavens. This beam would shine directly on my pelvis healing any areas that might be hindering my ability to conceive. After I became pregnant, I would visualize this beam of light shining on my belly creating a circle of protection. Be creative with your visualizations. There are no rules here, just what feels right and works for you.

I frequently looked in maternity shops or the maternity section of department stores. I had my whole maternity wardrobe planned out. When I saw pregnant women, rather than seeing them as some kind of threat, I would look at them in awe – what a miracle there is growing inside of them! It will be my turn – their pregnancy in no way threatened me. There *are* enough babies out there to go around. I looked at cribs and had my nursery planned. I kept all of these things to myself, of course, but in my mind, it was all a done deal. If you really want something you don't have, you need to actually behave as if you already have it. This helps it manifest in your life.

Vision Boards

One very helpful visualization technique is to make a vision board. I did this when I was trying to conceive and I believe it helped me attract my daughter into my life. Basically, all you need is some poster board or a bulletin board. Go out and get some magazines on babies, families, parenting and so on. Find pictures of adorable babies. One thing you could also do is put your own picture next to them. Place the pictures on the board in a collage type fashion and put it in a place where you will see it frequently. I knew one couple who was having trouble getting pregnant who made their refrigerator their vision board (and by the way, they now have two children without fertility treatments).

Don't be surprised if you actually dream about your future child at night. I did have a few dreams about my daughter when I was trying to conceive. According to Karen Melton, DH Psychology and Certified in Prenatal and Birth Therapy, "Dreams can also give advance information about the person coming to be born. The unborn child can also communicate with other receptive people in his/her environment – friends, family, co-workers. We are not all able to receive telepathic messages, and the unborn child will use who is available and receptive. Often in dreams or visitations the child will appear older, e.g. 3 or 6 years old, and multiple experiences may happen so that you really get to know your child before conception.

Many people dream before conception about what their child will look like at a certain age and when they get to that age they look exactly the way they did in the dream. Couples who have no intention of having a baby, or who have even had tubal ligations, will dream of a child wanting to be born to them, and this will have the effect of them changing their minds, even reversing surgery. Clearly these are not your ordinary everyday dreams, they have a clear and powerful message that can be life changing. At the least they offer the opportunity to fall in love with your child right from the beginning."[89]

I know many people use prayer instead of or with visualization and meditation. If prayer is part of your daily ritual and religion is an important part of your life, by all means, make it part of your fertility routine. Even though I said many prayers on the road to parenthood, I found visualization and meditation to be more empowering (and infertility can really test your faith). I've always felt prayer was asking for something vs. visualization and meditation were creating what you want. Do both if you choose.

If you need some fertility prayers, here are a few from the Christian perspective. I realize I have readers from all over the world with different religions, but these can be modified to fit your belief system.

Catholic Prayer

You know my deep desire for a child
A little one to love and to hold, to care for,
to cherish. Grant that my body may conceive
and give birth to a beautiful, healthy baby in
Your holy image.
Guide me in all my choices so that this
conception, my pregnancy and my baby's birth
are in line with Your will.
Heavenly Father and Holy Mother,
hear this prayer of my heart, mind and spirit.
Amen.[90]

---

[89] Melton, Karen. "Pre-conception and Conscious Conception." Heal Your Early Imprints. 30 July 2009. Web. 3 Mar. 2015. <www.healyourearlyimprints.com>.
[90] The Fertility Blessing - Prayers - Catholic Online. (n.d.). Retrieved March 4, 2015, from http://www.catholic.org/prayers/prayer.php?p=2985

Prayer for Fertility and Pregnancy

Lord bless us with a healthy child
Allow my body to conceive and carry a baby
Let this child be a symbol of our love as a couple
Let this child be born into our happy home

Help us let go of our disappointment and give us patience
We trust that you will send us a child when the time is right
We trust in your abundance
We are grateful for what you have given us and for what we have
We know that you are perfect in every way and our child will be a reflection of you and your love
Amen.

Prayer and Promise for A New Life

Blessed is this new life who will come into our family
We wait for your birth and we pray for your health
You are sent by God as a divine gift
We promise to love and cherish you throughout your life
We promise to raise you according to the word of God
We promise to protect and keep you from harm
Amen.

Prayer for Miscarriage

It is now that we reluctantly part
But I'll always keep you in my heart
Goodbye to what could have been
Goodbye until we meet again
Rest in peace with God and the Angels
Amen.

Changing Your Mindset and Clearing Your Mental Roadblocks Around Getting Pregnant

If you've been trying to get pregnant for over a year, you've probably built up a lot of sensitivity and negativity around the subject. Not only sensitivity and negativity, but a downright mental roadblock – and I mean that in every sense of the word. When you've failed to succeed at something for an extended period of time, you start to feel you are unworthy, incapable, and inferior to everyone else who has succeeded. When you want something so bad, and it's not coming, you try to force it into place. Believe me when I say babies can't be forced into anything. You need to change your mindset. Your body and mind need to be an open vessel. You need to prepare your body physically (with the steps I've outlined in this book) and you need to quit trying to hammer everything into place.

Babies come when *they're* good and ready not when you demand they come. You need to do the visualization and meditation exercises to show your future son or daughter they are welcome here with you, and you are ready and willing with open arms when they decide to make their journey. After your visualization and meditation, tell them that. Talk to them (out loud) and tell them you look forward to their arrival. Tell them you understand this is *their* decision to come and start their life with you. I truly believe babies select *you*, not the other way around. There is something very powerful about actually talking to your baby. It makes them *real*.

Have You Built Up Resistance?

Have you ever noticed things tend to come easily when you aren't trying so hard for them? Or when you're not trying at all? This seems to be a recurring theme in my life and it has taught me there really is such a thing as trying too hard. Perhaps all that "trying" is building up resistance to the very thing you want so much. After so much failure, you start focusing more on what you *don't* have. I know it's infuriating when people say, "just relax and it will happen". Probably the reason people say this so much is everyone seems to know a couple who had trouble conceiving, gave up, and got pregnant. The reason this happens is they lowered their resistance making room for success. You can't just want something, you need to *allow* it into your experience. The more negativity you have surrounding a particular subject, the more resistance you will build up. It is a really a slight shift in thinking that can make all the difference. You probably think it's an old wives tale that couples who adopt have a higher rate of natural conception afterwards. Actually, it's a complicated issue since you must exclude couples who have physical abnormalities that would make a natural pregnancy impossible. Although there are no statistics that claim there is a higher rate of couples who get pregnant naturally after adopting, I have read so many cases of this happening. I personally know two couples who experienced infertility, adopted and then got pregnant naturally. One couple adopted a baby from China, and during the process conceived naturally. As a result, they have two children the same age. They went on to conceive naturally again and now have three kids. The other couple was in my infertility support group. They adopted an older child, then got pregnant twice afterward and now have three children as well. Earlier, I mentioned that we're seeing an increasing number of women going through IVF who have one child and wind up getting pregnant naturally with their second. Now, do you think it might possibly have something to do with the release of their stress, anxiety and anger? It is my belief that couples who become pregnant after adopting experience the same phenomenon.

Know in your heart this *will* happen. There is no reason to be upset. Your baby is on the way. Don't force him or her to come before their time. You want your baby to be good and ready when he/she arrives. *Everything is right on schedule.* As a matter of fact, now that I have the benefit of hindsight, I'm glad I had my daughter when I did. If I had her when we first started trying to get pregnant, she'd be practically grown by now.

Defense Mechanisms

Many women who have gone through years of disappointment either with infertility or miscarriage start to put up their defense mechanisms by "not getting their hopes up" anymore. This is a mistake if you're trying to conceive. As hard as it might be, you need to dare to dream again. Even though I did have my defense mechanisms up from time to time, it really didn't stop the pain and disappointment each month when I didn't conceive. As far as miscarriage goes, it's devastating no matter what. Trying to conceive is a roller coaster ride that goes up and down at the beginning and end of each menstrual cycle. Of course you get your hopes up, how can you not? There is no sense in spending the time or energy in trying to convince yourself that you don't care. Just because you didn't get pregnant this month, it doesn't mean you won't get pregnant next month or the month after.

Maintain A Positive Mindset

Attracting the things you want in your life seems to happen when you maintain a positive mindset. You may be saying to yourself, "if I could just have a baby, I would be happy", it's really just the opposite. What you should say is, "If I could just be happy, I would have a baby"! Now, just for the record, I'm not a Pollyanna who always sees the glass half full (as a matter of fact, I usually expect the worst, and when something better happens, I am pleasantly surprised.) What I really mean is while you are waiting for your baby to come, keep yourself busy with things you enjoy. I really got into decorative painting (with nontoxic paint) during the years I was trying to conceive. I redecorated my sister's entire house and I made some beautiful painted floor cloths that now sit on our hardwood floors. Playing music you enjoy can turn a negative mood into a positive one. Only you know the things you truly enjoy. Think back to before you were on the "getting pregnant" rollercoaster. What did you enjoy doing? If you keep yourself busy with things you enjoy, believe me, your spirits will be uplifted and you will be more receptive. If you were a new soul ready to make the journey from conception to birth, wouldn't you prefer to come into a situation where everyone was happy and content? You need to create that environment for your baby.

How Can You Laugh At A Time Like This?

Probably the last thing you feel like doing while you're in the throes of infertility is laughing. Much has been written about the healing power of laughter and it can be an important factor in changing your mindset and lowering your resistance. Laughter can lower your blood pressure, reduce stress (and stress hormones), increase endorphins (natural painkillers) and strengthen the immune system. Best of all it's free and fun!

Has laughter ever been studied in regards to fertility? There was actually a study done in Israel on women undergoing IVF. Half of them were entertained by a clown for about 15 minutes after the embryos were transferred into their wombs. The routine included jokes, tricks, and magic and was performed on a one-to-one basis. The study sample included 219 patients (110 in the intervention group and 109 in the control group). There were no significant differences between the groups regarding age. The pregnancy rate in the intervention group was 36.4%, compared with 20.2% in the control group. Researchers thought "laughter may have an effect on the embryo-uterine interplay through neuroendocrine pathways or non-ovarian stress reduction, augmenting uterine receptivity".[91]

Although this study was done on women undergoing IVF, I can't help but believe that the beneficial effect of laughter can help women who are trying to conceive naturally too. How can you laugh at a time like this? You just have to figure out what tickles your funny bone. For me, watching the television show where people send in their silly home videos was a guaranteed laugh. Sometimes I'd have tears running down my face I would laugh so hard. Try it! I didn't always feel like laughing, but I'd start watching and I couldn't contain myself! Many cable channels play the reruns at all hours and you can find almost anything online, so it's pretty easy to find at least one episode per day. It's those belly laughs that make you cry that are especially healing and cathartic.

---

[91] Friedler, Shevach et al.,The effect of medical clowning on pregnancy rates after in vitro fertilization and embryo transfer, Fertility and Sterility , Volume 95 , Issue 6 , 2127 - 2130

Go Ahead and Have A Good Cry

I know I just said to maintain a positive mindset and to have a good belly laugh, however, crying can be good for your emotional health as well. I shed many tears on the road to parenthood and I must say, I did feel better after a good cathartic cry. Tears may be involved in the elimination of harmful substances and toxins from the body. They also help to regulate emotions. Every now and then it just feels good to let it all out, and not feel like you have to be so strong. I believe you need to release those negative emotions which creep up from time to time. It's hard to be positive when you're all bottled up. I'm not saying you should stay in a negative place, but you do need to acknowledge these feelings, release them and move on. As a matter of fact, I had a major cry session right before I conceived my daughter. I actually screamed to the point that I wondered if my neighbors could hear me. Even though this was tough, I felt really peaceful afterward. I can't help but think that this emotional (and physical) release helped move my body to a place where it could accept and hold on to a successful pregnancy.

Acknowledge the Positive Aspects Of Your Life

Do *not* focus on your infertility. Look at all the positive aspects of your life and write these in a journal. Even though your struggle to get pregnant has been grueling, has it brought positive things into your life? For me, it forced me to confront some of my past demons (see my chapter, "How I Became My Own Therapist") which has helped me not only be a better parent, but also a better wife and better overall person. It led me to be much healthier by reducing my stress level and it changed the way I eat (I still eat just as healthy now). Going through this experience has also shown me I am a very strong and capable person with more patience than I thought I could ever muster up. Writing all these things down is very helpful because when you start to slip into negativity, you can go back and review what you've written.

De-clutter Your Life & Environment

Another important piece of the puzzle is to de-clutter your life and your environment. To de-clutter your life, ask yourself if you are doing things out of obligation. Have you said "yes" to things that you couldn't say "no" to? Part of keeping a positive mindset is doing things you enjoy. It's your life and this is your time. Don't waste it out of obligation.

De-cluttering your environment involves going through your home and getting rid of the old to make room for the new. Is your house or apartment full of junk you aren't using? Take a day every week and start sifting through your stuff. I always use the "one year rule". If I haven't used something or worn something for an entire year (ok, maybe a year and a half), then I get rid of it. I always donate it to a not for profit organization or second hand store where someone will really benefit from it. It really is a relief to have a de-cluttered home. You think more clearly, you become more efficient and you have more of a sense of well-being. If you have a room in your home you've designated as a nursery, make sure it's de-cluttered as well. I think we all have the temptation to use spare rooms as dumping grounds, but it's not very welcoming to your new baby. We had a spare room that just sat empty for years (I used to sort the laundry in it). When we got serious about having a baby, I actually decorated the room (not in baby décor, but in flowery fabric) just to have an inviting environment. You'll be surprised how much better you feel when your home is in order. See also my "Alternative Techniques" chapter for more on feng shui to create a welcoming home for your baby.

Chapter 7
Join a Support Group

After everything I'd been through I finally thought a support group would help me out. One reason I thought about joining a support group was I could make new friends who did not have children (many people my age were so wrapped up with their families, they really did not have time to devote to their friends). When I quit working in the corporate world, it seemed my social circle shrunk significantly. I was teaching at a community college, but since I was part-time and practically an independent contractor, I didn't have a lot of one on one contact with my co-workers. I also wanted to make a connection with others who ate, drank, and slept getting pregnant like I did. Believe it or not, there is some evidence that support group attendance by women who are trying to conceive actually does increase live pregnancy rates. [92]

I had heard of a non-profit infertility support organization through my previous RE's office called "Resolve". I didn't pay much attention to the flyers I saw there when I was going through fertility treatments because I thought I had no use for a support group (in retrospect I should have joined back then). I was now ready. I looked up the organization on-line to find the number for the local

---

[92]Domar AD, Clapp D, Slawsby E, Kessel B, Orav J, Freizinger M.,The impact of group psychological interventions on distress in infertile women, Health Psychol. 2000 Nov;19(6):568-75.

chapter (I believe every state has one – type "infertility support" on your search engine). I called the number and received a call back from the chapter president. She told me the group met at least one time per month and sometimes more. I got on the mailing list and attended my first meeting in August.

I was really nervous to attend the meeting. I was afraid everyone else would know each other and I'd be somewhat of an outsider. The meetings were held at the home of a group member and everyone would take turns hosting the meetings. When I arrived, I felt very much at home. Before the meeting started, everyone was freely talking and I immediately felt like one of the group. Many people knew each other very well, but there were other new members like myself.

When the meeting got started, we went around the room and everyone told their stories of how long they'd been trying to get pregnant, what treatments they had gone through, and anything else they wanted to discuss. My first meeting had about ten people but some meetings had as many as 13 or as few as 5. Everyone had their own story to tell. Many had already gone through IVF with no success or succeeded only to miscarry. Some were trying to get pregnant with Clomid or inseminations. Some had premature ovarian failure and were looking at using donor eggs. Some were taking the natural route like me. I was the oldest, but not by much. There were others that were over 40, but some younger women had gone through premature menopause. A few had male factor infertility and were looking at using donor sperm or ICSI (where they inject one sperm into the egg).

Most women were in their late 30's and 40's and they all started nodding when I spoke about the "infertility profile".

Here are some factors we all seem to have in common - see if they apply to you:
1. Career Oriented - enjoy being in a high ranking position
2. Delayed marriage and childbearing to pursue career or other personal interests
3. Somewhat of a perfectionist
4. Perhaps had a less than perfect upbringing or volatile relationship with parents or family
5. Approval Addict (the need for others to recognize that you're doing a good job)
6. Hard worker - always meet deadlines
7. Eventually succeed in everything you do (except getting pregnant - at least for the time being!)

It was so nice to be in a room full of people who were just like me. Joining a support group reduces your feelings of being some kind of freak. When you know there are others struggling with the same thing, you realize infertility is quite common. Infertility can also be a very isolating experience because you feel left behind when friends, family members, and other acquaintances are having children. There is something very comforting about the unconditional acceptance you feel with a group of others who are just like you. Support groups also give you the opportunity to take the focus off yourself. It is really quite a relief to help others when you're struggling with something so all consuming. Additionally, if you've decided to keep your infertility private, a support group gives you a safe place to "let it all out".

I know there those who see support groups as "misery loves company pity parties". It's truly not that way. We would talk about doctors, herbs, natural treatments, books, past members who succeeded, and much more. I always looked forward to our meetings and it was nice to have a new social circle of friends who I had so much in common with.

If there is not a support group in your area, think about joining an on-line support group. As I mentioned above, if you type "infertility support" on your search engine, you should be able to find a number of online chat rooms and support forums. You should also be able to find out if there is a group that meets in person in your area. I think it was very helpful to attend meetings in person, but if it's not possible for you to do this, or if you prefer staying completely anonymous, consider joining an on-line group.

One interesting thing they discussed at my first meeting was the group leader (who was simply a volunteer) always became pregnant (I've also heard this frequently happens with on-line groups!) I tucked that in the back of my mind. I was a good organizer, and I thought I would volunteer to be the group leader the next time there was an opening.

I religiously attended every meeting. Sure enough, the group leader became pregnant. She had previously asked another group member to take over the group, but I told the new group leader I would be happy to be a co-leader with her. The new leader had PCOS (polycystic ovarian syndrome). She and her husband finally decided to try IVF at least once. This was a big step for her since she wanted to stick with the all-natural route. Her IVF cycle was going to be the month after she became the group leader. I had a strong suspicion she was going to succeed, so I knew I would be taking over the group. Sure enough, she became pregnant on the first IVF try. I guess there really was something to it – the group leader *did* become pregnant!

I took over the group shortly thereafter. I guess it was my years working as a manager, but I really loved being an organizer and a leader. It was also nice to feel like I was doing *something* – even if it benefited other people rather than myself. I kept the group going strong and I saw a number of members succeed and move on. It had now been a year since I joined the group and I was still not pregnant. My husband and I held firm on our commitment not go through any more fertility treatments. I was 43 and I had another birthday coming up. There was actually one woman older than me in the group now. She was 45.

As much as I enjoyed being in the group and being a group leader, the constant disappointment of not getting pregnant every month was starting to wear on me. I was watching others in the group get pregnant, and I was beginning to wonder if I had just gotten too old. I decided if I was not pregnant by my 44th birthday, I needed to quit. I was feeling the need to move on with my life. I felt the stark realization that I might never succeed was starting to sink in. I didn't know if I had the energy anymore to maintain a positive attitude and my spirits began to plummet. I was tired of thinking about getting pregnant and I made a very tough decision that in September (my 44th birthday was in October) I was going to resign from the group and move on to "childfree".

During the August meeting, I announced my decision. I told the group I would host the next meeting in September but I needed a new volunteer to take over the group. In many ways it felt good to have finally come to a firm decision and to be moving on to something new. That doesn't mean it was easy, as I mentioned earlier, there was one day I was home alone and I just screamed at the top of my lungs – I don't know who I was screaming to – maybe God, maybe the universe, maybe myself. I had done all the right things, I stayed healthy, I visualized, I meditated, I had actually gotten pregnant 6 times (see my chapter on "My Experience with Recurrent Miscarriage") ----*but no baby.*

After my decision to move on to childfree, I thought about trying to find other friends who were not on the "mommy" track or perhaps others my age who had older children and had time to devote to friendships. I really think it helps your transition to childfree if you're not constantly associating with others who are doing the family thing. I first looked at reconnecting with a few old friends of mine, one had stayed single and never had children and another was divorced and never had children. I also had a sister who stayed single and had many single or married friends with no children. I thought about joining a recreation group with my husband – something just to meet others who had either made the decision not to have children (childfree by choice) or others who were like us and were unable to have kids.

My last support group meeting was bittersweet. It was the end of my dream to become a parent, but in some ways it was exciting to be letting go of the constant disappointment and to be moving on with my life. I told the group I would miss them and I wished them all the best of luck *and I really meant it.* I apologized for breaking the group leader winning streak since I was the first leader I knew of who was going to quit without success. One of the hardest parts of letting go was I had to admit to myself I failed. This was the first time in my life all the hard work and perseverance just did not pay off. I also felt my "internal compass" was broken. I was so sure I would get pregnant, but I didn't. Even though it was time to move on, I still had this unfinished feeling like something still might happen but I couldn't take it any longer. It just wasn't fair, but I had to remind myself of all of the positive things infertility had brought to my life. I was healthier than I had ever been, it was the reason I quit a high pressure job I didn't like anyway, and I confronted a lot of issues in my life that were holding me back.

At the end of my last meeting, we all hugged and said goodbye. I was truly moving on and I was okay with it. I felt a little bad about leaving since these people had been my main social circle for the last year. But part of moving on was to get away from the "getting pregnant" scene and all these people were in the thick of it. It was like I was moving out of town but I was moving to a different phase in my life. Good-bye to my dream of being a parent, good-bye to my period calendar, good-bye to the infertile world, good-bye to the constant disappointment. Whew! What a relief!

Two weeks later, I found out I was pregnant.

Go figure.

Chapter 8
All Stressed Up and Going Nowhere

Many women who experience infertility are career oriented and put having children on the back burner. Although getting on the career track is certainly a legitimate life choice, it often leads to getting married at an older age and trying to have children even later. On top of all that, career oriented women have increased their stress load as much if not more than their male counterparts. I know for me, being a woman in the corporate world meant I had to work harder and shine brighter than most of the men in my position just to get the same respect.

I know you've heard it all before, "reduce your stress level if you want to get pregnant". The reason you hear this so much is physiologically, stress *can* affect your fertility. Cortisol, a hormone secreted during times of stress, can affect ovulation and/or contribute to shorter menstrual cycles. Additionally, stress may be a contributing factor in miscarriage (stress hormones have even been found in miscarried fetuses). My message to you is you actually have to make the changes in your life that are going to *really* make a difference. If you're in a high stress job, this is the time to ask yourself some tough questions about your priorities. When I was right out of college, I got my first high-stress position as a manager. It was a bit of a head trip to be in a well-paying powerful job, however it started me on a downward spiral in terms of my overall health.

Whether you're in a management position or not, many jobs out there have incredibly high levels of stress. When there is a downturn in the economy, corporations downsize and those who are left have to pick up the slack. I went through this a number of times – I was one of the survivors, but I'm beginning to think I would have been better off being laid off! The Women's Reproductive Health Study conducted in California found that women in stressful jobs had twice the risk of short cycle length than women in in less stressful jobs. Psychological job stress and social support at work were assessed with 13 questions that concerned stress related job characteristics, four were combined to measure job demand, five were combined to measure job control, and four were combined to measure social support at work. "One possible explanation of work-related stress and increased risk for short cycle length is that luteinizing hormone secretion has been inhibited by an increase in corticotropin-releasing hormone or glucocorticoids."[93] Back when I worked in the corporate world, I did experience shorter cycles which I was able to lengthen after changing my lifestyle.

Additionally, another study found that women who work alternating shifts suffered menstrual disruption, which can cause fertility problems.[94] In my chapter, "Preventing Miscarriage", I also talk about how shift work can lead to a higher incidence of pregnancy loss.

Everyone has their own way of dealing with stress and, for most, it's an unhealthy way. For me, I kept a very calm

---

[93] Fenster, L., Waller, K., Chen, J., Hubbard, A., Windham, G., Elkin, E., & Swan, S. (1998). Psychological Stress in the Workplace and Menstrual Function. American Journal of Epidemiology, 149(2), 127-134.

[94] Fertility experts say night shift workers 'more likely to suffer miscarriages' (2013, July 9). Retrieved March 30, 2015, from http://www.uhs.nhs.uk/AboutTheTrust/Newsandpublications/Latestnews/2013/Fertility-experts-say-night-shift-workers-more-likely-to-suffer-miscarriages.aspx

exterior (employees would ask me how I stayed so calm all the time), but what didn't show on the outside was the gut wrenching turmoil I felt in the pit of my stomach (and in my reproductive system!) I personally know my stress manifested itself in uterine fibroids and endometriosis. I've known women who had terrible pain with their periods and once they quit their jobs, and changed their lifestyle, the pain literally went away. I look back now at the days when I was on the career track and I truly can't even believe what a crazy stressful time it was. There is *no way* I could go back and do that again now, nor would I want to. When you're stuck in the rat race, you have no concept of what a healthy lifestyle looks like.

You need to be completely honest with yourself about your ability to deal with stress. Even if you take classes in stress management (which basically deal with your reaction to stress vs. the stress itself), if you can't completely implement what you've learned, you may still be in the same boat. I finally came to the conclusion I needed to get away from my high stress job and I made the decision to quit before we started our IVF cycles (I guess my fertility treatments were good for something, because I probably would have never quit otherwise!) My strong work ethic would not allow me to cut back the way I needed to, so leaving was the only way I could ensure I would reduce my stress level. This was a *major* life decision for me because I was making good money and I had excellent benefits.

Do You Really Have To Work?

Most people are afraid to quit their jobs, but you need to examine your finances closely to figure out if there is a way to make things work on one income. Yes, you need to adjust your spending habits, but I found that once I quit my job, I really didn't spend as much money. I didn't have to buy a wardrobe, I ate lunch at home, I spent less on gas, etc. You also might have to examine certain luxuries you can live without. Again, it's a matter of priorities. I've known people who moved to smaller homes and sold possessions to make it on one income. For me, having a child was *absolutely* my number one priority. Giving up my career was also difficult because I had so much of my self-worth wrapped up in it and it was part of my identity. You can always get another job, but you may not have another opportunity to have a child. If you're over 40, you really need to make those changes *now*, because 10 years from now, a biological child may not be possible.

One added benefit of quitting my job was I was able to completely relax. I literally had not had more than 2 weeks off in a row in 19 years. Life was so much more enjoyable when I didn't have to answer to employees, a boss, or a corporation for every minute of the day. It also freed up my mind and allowed me to get rid of the negativity that builds up day after day in a high stress job. I started to meditate and was able to have a clear enough mind to visualize a healthy pregnancy from conception to childbirth.

If you quit your job, you're in a better position of being able to clean up your diet. When you eat at home, you have the time to prepare a healthy meal. I know I would not have been able to eat as well as I did if I was gulping down my lunch between crises like I did at work. You're also able to get healthy exercise (again, not too much), but you have the time to go for nice leisurely walks and enjoy just being outdoors.

If you *absolutely (emphasis on absolutely)* have to have your income to survive, do an objective assessment of what is demanded of you on your job. Can you eliminate or get help with some of the more stressful aspects of your job? If you're a manager, can you take a different non-management position? Do you need to look at working for a different company that has a less stressful atmosphere? Can you work part-time? Perhaps you could find a way to work from home (at least you could eat healthier and avoid office politics.)

Quitting my job, in my opinion, was one of the major factors in my successful pregnancy. I don't miss it and I've never regretted it. Although I feel it is the combination of things I listed in this book that led to my success, I don't think I could have succeeded while working in the corporate pressure cooker. I know how hard it is to give up the workplace "golden shackles" (i.e. money, power, perks), but don't you want more out of life? I certainly did! If you think money and possessions make you happy, think again. When you have this wonderful miracle of life you love with all your heart and soul, you realize how empty a life of climbing the corporate ladder can be. Besides, babies don't really care how much money you have. They simply want your love and attention. Now that I have my daughter, I'm so absorbed with taking care of her, I'm much less materialistic. I buy things now because I *need* them, not because I'm trying to impress somebody. I really don't care how big my house is or what kind of car I drive.

Driven By Deadlines?

Once I quit my job, I found I was more patient. When you're in the career mode, you always feel like things have to be done by some deadline. Living your life on deadlines and schedules isn't compatible with getting pregnant. I've actually known people going through fertility treatments who had a target date for when they were going to get pregnant. This led to double the frustration and disappointment if their cycle was cancelled or if their procedure failed. I even knew a woman who said, "I definitely want to get pregnant before my sister who is getting married next month." This is not a contest! When you've failed to get pregnant month after month, it can be devastating when someone else (who isn't even trying that hard) gets pregnant before you. I had a cousin who had two children and completed her entire family all within the time I was trying to get pregnant. Everyone's situation is different. The feeling like you're losing the race adds unnecessary pressure to the mix. I think there's a temptation to feel like others are trying to "rub your nose in it" when they get pregnant before you. It's hard to painstakingly watch while they get on with their life and you're stuck in "infertility quicksand". Believe me when I say *none* of this will matter after you succeed.

We've all heard people talk about their biological clock which is frankly quite annoying. I've even heard 29 year olds say their biological clock is screaming! *Oh please!* If I had been concerned about this proverbial biological clock, I would have given up before I ever had a chance to succeed (if anyone's biological clock had already gone off, it was mine!) I can't say enough how completely unproductive it is to compare yourself to others. Setting deadlines for getting pregnant or anything else for that matter creates undue stress if you can't achieve it within your specified timeframe.

Stress From Approval Addiction

Are you an approval addict? I have to admit, I was. This is one reason I wanted to climb the corporate ladder. Every time I got a promotion, it said to me, *"You've done such a good job".* Those were the moments I lived for. The down side is the moment someone significant in your life expresses disapproval, you immediately fall down in the dumps. Having someone else responsible for your self-esteem serves no purpose except to add to your stress.

Also along the lines of approval addition, at one time, I felt I was a failure in the eyes of my peers. Whenever I ran into someone I grew up with, or went to a high school reunion, I felt like I was less than everyone else because I had not achieved the "American Dream". I felt people took pity on me because I didn't have children. I had to remind myself people were not looking down on me, just like I don't look down on other women who don't have children. I remember a saying I heard once which always brings comfort when I fall into the trap of worrying about what other people think:

In your 20's, you care what *everyone* thinks
In your 30's you don't care what *anyone* thinks
In your 40's, you realize *nobody* was thinking about you anyway!

Evaluate Your Social Structure

Have you filled your life with people you feel good around? There are plenty of positive people in the world, you don't need to be around those that bring you down or leave you feeling drained or upset. There actually have been studies that show people with a strong supportive social structure live longer and report being happier. This is one good reason to join a support group. I recall when I worked in the corporate world, I was forced to deal with coworkers who were very negative and difficult to work with adding to an already stressful situation.

Having an animal to love has also been shown to reduce stress and lower blood pressure in some people. Maybe you need cuddly pet if you don't already have one. If you get a pet, make sure it's "kid friendly." I had a cat during my first IVF cycle, but she was very elderly and died before my second IVF. I was unable to get another cat due to my husband's allergies but curling up with a lovable pet was very comforting during the tough times.

I noticed a number of positive changes when I finally was able to relax and remove all the stressors in my life. The skin on my face finally cleared up! I never had a real acne problem, but my chin always had some kind of breakout going on (another possible indicator of hormonal imbalance). I also found that I was just a nicer person when I wasn't carrying the weight of the world around on my shoulders twenty-four hours a day, seven days per week (as I did when I was working full-time). Stress makes you irritable and can make you difficult to live with.

Chapter 9
How I Became My Own Therapist

Most of us who have delayed childbearing have done so for many reasons, but I would venture to guess we didn't have the ideal upbringing or we had it down right rough. This has led us to put having children low on our priority list (or not on the list at all) because we didn't have a favorable impression of family life. You may have spent a good deal of your adult life feeling like this is *my* time – I don't have enough left in me to take care of someone else.

This is one of the most important things to go back and examine *now*. The reason is, whether you are aware of it or not, you are carrying your past anger, resentments and hurts around with you. Your past is affecting your actions, your health, your thinking, and ultimately, your ability to get pregnant. If you have spent much of your life not wanting children (or thinking you didn't want them), it only makes sense it's going to take a little work to change some of your automatic thoughts. Your body may be holding on to your previous desire not to have children. The good news is *you* are in control. Your mind is the captain of the ship – it can tell your body what to do.

When I attended my high school reunions my classmates without exception said to me "You were true to your word, you said you didn't want kids, and you don't have any". That was always an eye opener for me, because I was trying to get pregnant at the time of my 20 year reunion (although I did not share this with anyone). It reminded me of one of the big reasons why I was having so much trouble getting pregnant. I had started my negative thinking about having children way back in high school. I knew it was going to take some time to reverse this whole mindset.

Because I had spent so much of my life not wanting kids I had to ask myself why. I honestly believe most people have a natural desire or instinct to procreate. When you spend a good part of your life going against something that should be so natural, there's got to be some significance to it. You need to do more than just scratch the surface, you need to go down deep and confront any negativity you have toward your family (the one you grew up with) or anyone else who is a big part of your life. Many women I've met who were struggling with infertility had very similar stories about their upbringing.

According to Karen Melton, DH Psychology and Certified in Prenatal and Birth Therapy,

"Pre-conception is an ideal time to be thinking about and assessing all aspects of your life and the changes you may want to make before you become pregnant. These changes could be to your career, emotional/psychological, physical and health, in your home or the location of your home, and in your relationship with each other. Having a baby is going to create huge changes in your lives, which you will have to manage in the midst of sleep deprivation – loss of freedom, changes in your sexual life, etc. These changes can be overwhelming, unless you are prepared."

"The kind of womb, and family, that your baby comes into is going to have a profound impact upon her whole life. You can both prepare for your new baby by healing:

- Trauma's based in your sexuality/pelvic area such as sexual abuse
- Un-grieved or unresolved prior abortions, miscarriages or stillbirth.
- Anything else you are holding in your womb – women often hold stress and trauma in their Pelvic Bowl area, and especially in their reproductive system.
- Unresolved conception, womb, birth and bonding traumas from your own journey's here, that are specifically likely to affect the way you bring your own children into life.
- Relationship issues you have with each other, particularly around becoming parents, parenting styles, and unresolved parenting and ancestral issues from both sides of your families.

The benefits of exploring your own conception, womb, birth and bonding experiences are enormous for both your baby, and for the impact they will have on your own lives individually and as parents. The quality of the conscious parenting you will be able to offer her/him right from the very beginning is priceless. The parenting you received will shape the parenting you will give, even if you consciously don't want it to! Many of our formative experiences are deeply unconscious and still strongly influencing our lives. You can, with awareness and consciousness, make choices about what you want to pass on to your children.

You don't have to be perfect to be a good parent. A commitment to your own ongoing healing and consciousness, and to developing and maintaining a good relationship, is a wonderful foundation for parenthood. Develop good communication skills, keep your love alive and be willing to plumb your own depths to create fulfilling lives for your whole family. If you bond with your baby before conception, and throughout pregnancy, and birthing and communicate with her/him throughout, you can mitigate many of life's stresses and trauma's for your child."[95]

In my case, I still had a lot of issues with my parents, my mother in particular. I was quite angry with her for never showing me any kind of love. She clothed me, fed me, educated me, brought me to church, and from the outside everything looked fine. The problem is I never felt loved, I had the feeling like I was an unwanted guest in the house and I should make myself as scarce as possible. My middle sister (I was the youngest) got her attention by always being the helper to the point that my mother delegated all of the parenting to her. I deeply resented this because even at a very young age, this communicated to me I was unworthy of my mother's love. As I got older, I started hating my mother for this and I would constantly pick fights with her. I guess deep down I just wanted her to tell me she loved me and give me some individual attention. I cannot remember even one instance of her hugging me or telling me she loved me. In contrast, I probably tell my daughter I love her twenty times a day if not more! I knew I could get my mother's attention by acting out, so I did, *frequently.* This ultimately backfired by driving her even further away from me.

I led a very lonely existence at home. I almost had a feeling of hopelessness because I truly felt nobody cared about me. I would frequently stay after school or go over my friends' houses because they had parents who took an interest in them (and me!) If I ever joined a team of any sort, I always had to hitch a ride with a teammate. Again, I felt unworthy of having my own parent there. The one time my mother was assigned to bring the soda pop after a softball game, she didn't show up (the game ended early

---

[95] Melton, Karen. "Pre-conception and Conscious Conception." Heal Your Early Imprints. 30 July 2009. Web. 3 Mar. 2015. <www.healyourearlyimprints.com>.

and she was late). *God forbid she should actually stay and watch the game!* I was humiliated, embarrassed, but *not* surprised. I was always the last on the list and this only confirmed it.

My father was a workaholic businessman. He was a very good provider, and he saw this as his sole responsibility in the family. I do appreciate now that he supported the family so well, but in retrospect, his absence only added to the isolation and loneliness I felt as a child and it added to my mother's workload. In my parents' generation, men frequently were let off the hook when it came to raising children. I guess, even now, I don't hold him responsible for my lack of parenting (even though I probably should).

When you're a young child or a teenager, you don't have the wisdom or the insight to understand why things are the way they are. You tend to think everything is your fault and you don't know how to change it. I knew my parents and sisters labeled me the difficult child, and I certainly lived up to my reputation. It wasn't until I was much older that I was able to clearly see how I was caught in a vicious cycle. I wanted to be a better person at home, but I was so busy trying to get what was rightfully mine (in terms of attention), that I couldn't focus on anything else. Kansas State University has published this questionnaire[96] to help you assess your own situation. If you find yourself answering "yes" to over half of the following questions (like I did), you likely have some long-term effects of living in a dysfunctional family:

1. Do you find yourself needing approval from others to feel good about yourself?

---

[96] Dysfunctional Families: Recognizing and Overcoming Their Effects. (n.d.). Retrieved April 2, 2015, from http://www.k-state.edu/counseling/topics/relationships/dysfunc.html

2. Do you agree to do more for others than you can comfortably accomplish?
3. Are you perfectionistic?
4. Or do you tend to avoid or ignore responsibilities?
5. Do you find it difficult to identify what you're feeling?
6. Do you find it difficult to express feelings?
7. Do you tend to think in all-or-nothing terms?
8. Do you often feel lonely even in the presence of others?
9. Is it difficult for you to ask for what you need from others?
10. Is it difficult for you to maintain intimate relationships?
11. Do you find it difficult to trust others?
12. Do you tend to hang on to hurtful or destructive relationships?
13. Are you more aware of others' needs and feelings than your own?
14. Do you find it particularly difficult to deal with anger or criticism?
15. Is it hard for you to relax and enjoy yourself?
16. Do you find yourself feeling like a "fake" in your academic or professional life?
17. Do you find yourself waiting for disaster to strike even when things are going well in your life?
18. Do you find yourself having difficulty with authority figures?

Journaling

Part of my pregnancy protocol was using a journal to confront all or most of the issues I was still struggling with from my past and my dysfunctional family. Journaling has been found to have long-term health benefits when used to confront traumatic and upsetting experiences.[97] I was fairly certain that my inability to have a child was somehow

---

[97] Karen A. Baikie, Kay Wilhelm, Emotional and physical health benefits of expressive writing, DOI: 10.1192/apt.11.5.338 Published 31 August 2005

connected to my own lack of parenting and my resentment which I was still carrying around with me. I would write these issues in my journal and then I would use a technique of responding to each issue from my parents' point of view. I would also think about what I wanted them to say to me and I would include this in their response. I did not discuss any of this with my mother (and my father passed away many years ago.) I suppose I could have actually discussed each issue with my mother, since she's still living, but honestly, I didn't have the desire to get into a big confrontation. Additionally, sometimes my mother doesn't express herself well. She'll say one thing but mean another. I knew in my heart what she would say if she had the ability to know what was going on inside of me and if she had the ability to talk in a way that would preserve my feelings. I know my mother would not intentionally hurt me, but she could sometimes be brutally candid – probably because she didn't have the verbal skills to rephrase things tactfully.

An example of what I would write in my journal is below:

Issue: My mother showered my sisters with love and attention but ignored me. This made me feel like a second class citizen in the household and unworthy of love. My mother's eyes would light up when my sisters came in the room and she would always be talking favorably about them to her friends. She rarely said anything about me. When my mother looked at me, her face would be blank. No smile, no glimmer of approval, just a cold stare and sometimes a downright frown or glare. My mother delegated her parenting to my middle sister. This showed me I wasn't good enough to actually have love and attention from a *real* parent.

My mother's point of view: "I was raising three children, working full time, trying to cook, keep the house up inside and out, and keep everyone on their schedules – I was under a tremendous amount of stress. I know I should have shown you more love and given you more attention, but by the time you came along, I felt like I was always on the edge of losing control. My hectic schedule overtook my life and unfortunately you took the brunt of it. I am deeply sorry. I shouldn't have relied so much on your sister to raise you, but she was always there to step in and I took advantage of that. It was unfair to both of you. I know I was the source of your unhappiness. If I had given you more attention you wouldn't have felt the need to act out which would have helped me love you. I was the adult. I was the one with the problem, not you."

Responding to each issue from the *other* person's point of view helps you to see there are two sides to every story. I honestly feel people don't intentionally mistreat you. They have their own issues which affect their behavior. Even if you were the one to act out (as I did), you have to tell yourself that your behavior was a result of your situation. You did the best you could under the circumstances and most likely, people who mistreated you did the best they could do at the time. It is so helpful to acknowledge this because it sets you free from the weight of your past.

I continued writing in my journal about every issue I felt anger or hurt about. Don't think you can do this in one day…it may take weeks or months to dig deep down and pull up things that have been festering. You may find yourself getting quite emotional as you do this. I would frequently cry and feel angry – once I even screamed (alone of course), but all this is good – it's better outside of you than inside.

Examine Your Fears and Anxieties About Getting Pregnant

One thing I had to admit to myself was I had a lot of anxiety about getting pregnant. *What if something went wrong with the baby? What if there were complications during the delivery? What if I couldn't be a good mother? What if I turned out to be fat and frumpy the rest of my life? What if I couldn't ever get a good night's sleep again? What if, what if, what if...*

It's hard to be honest about your anxieties especially when you're trying so hard to get pregnant. You almost feel guilty for having any thought to the contrary. I had a number of miscarriages prior to my successful pregnancy and I'd be lying if I didn't say there was a tiny piece of me that was relieved when I did. It's *really* hard to admit that, but confronting my fears about getting pregnant and the guilt I felt about how I might be responsible for my miscarriages was crucial to my success. I would write each one of these issues in my journal and I would thoroughly examine each one. Then I would write an objective response to each issue to dispel the fear and anxiety. This brought my thoughts back down to reality. Here are a few examples:

Issue: "What if something goes wrong with the baby (especially at my age)?"

Rational Response: "Even though there is a higher incidence of chromosomal abnormalities in babies born to older women, it is still quite rare. There's no reason to think I will have an abnormal baby. There are a number of screening tests they can do to look for abnormalities (i.e. AFP, Amniocentesis, Ultrasound, etc.) These tests will put my mind at ease. Every woman who is pregnant faces these fears and somehow they all pull through. Most women have perfectly healthy babies, and even if they don't, they find the strength to deal with it."

Issue: "What if I turn out to be fat and frumpy the rest of my life? I've spent most of my life (since about 11 years old) doing everything I can to stay in shape and maintain a healthy weight. There was a time when getting fat was a fate worse than death! I still carry some of that around with me. Now, here I am, trying to get pregnant, volunteering to gain a previously unthinkable amount of weight and stretching body beyond the point of no return!"

Rational Response: "Yes, there are plenty of women who never lose their "baby" weight, but there are also plenty of women who do. As a matter of fact, I know a number of women who look better *after* they had their kids than before. There's no reason to think I won't maintain a healthy diet and exercise routine after I have my baby. I'll probably be more motivated than ever to stay in shape. My fertility diet has taught me how to eat in a way that is completely inconsistent with gaining weight. I know this is in my control and I know my attitude about health is so solid that I'll be successful in reestablishing my pre-pregnancy routine."

Issue: "If I get pregnant again, I'll just have another miscarriage. What makes me think the next pregnancy is going to be any different from all the others? I must be unworthy of having a baby. Maybe I'm being punished for something I did in my past."

Rational Response: "Miscarriages are quite common. I'm always surprised how many people tell my they've miscarried at least once. Even though having repeatedly

How I Became My Own Therapist

miscarried may be a risk factor for future miscarriages (at least statistically), I know many people who've had at least three miscarriages and went on to have successful pregnancies afterwards. I even know of a woman who had nine miscarriages and eventually succeeded in having a baby! Anything is possible!

None of the doctors have been able to tell me with certainty why I have miscarried. My pregnancy protocol will help me strengthen my reproductive system and balance my hormones so the next one *will* endure. I *am* worthy of having a child! I have the wisdom and the patience to be a wonderful parent. I am not being punished. I have led a good life and I've treated others with consideration and respect."

Go through all of your fears and anxieties and come up with logical and realistic responses to each of them. It is helpful to imagine yourself talking to a friend who had these concerns. What would you say to them to put their mind at ease?

Another option you might consider is to go to a therapist or counselor. There are therapists who work with infertile couples (one or both of you). If you choose this option, be sure to find a therapist who wholeheartedly embraces your decision to embark on a natural path to pregnancy no matter what your age. I did not go to a therapist because I wasn't sure I could completely open up to a stranger. I personally feel I was quite successful with the journaling technique. Furthermore, we had previously spent so much money on fertility treatments that I didn't want to drain any more financial resources. Many insurance plans are a bit "sketchy" when it comes to paying for counseling so it could be more of a private pay situation. Do what works for you, but at the very least, go through the journaling exercise. It will help you in all aspects of your life, not just getting pregnant.

Chapter 10
Putting it All Together
A Typical Day On My Pregnancy Protocol

I've included quite a bit of information here and it may seem somewhat overwhelming. So let's go through a typical day on my pregnancy protocol to put it all together. Before embarking on this protocol, some things you may want to do in preparation which I've included in previous chapters:
Journaling to confront mental roadblocks
Emotional Freedom Technique
Rearranging your home using feng shui design principles to create "baby chi"
Create your vision board

8:00am

Wake up preferable after 8- 9 hours of sleep (if you choose to establish your ovulation pattern by the BBT method, take your temperature)

8:15am

Drink 2 glasses of water (as mentioned earlier, this is based on the Ayurvedic water treatment which recommends up to 6 glasses, but I usually just had two)

8:30-9:30am

Take an alternating ice/hot bath (only the first half of your cycle before ovulation).

9:30- 10:00am

Drink Fertility Tea. Remember to wait a full hour after drinking the water in the morning before consuming anything else. Eat a banana and 8oz glass of soy milk sweetened with a little chocolate (many days I would also eat a couple of servings of broccoli or cauliflower (yes...in the morning!). Other options instead of soymilk include a wheatgrass or spirulina smoothie and/or a serving of my juiced vegetables.

10:00-11:00am

Take a walk outside and let the sun hit my retina. If it's warm enough, let the sun also hit your skin for vitamin D (this can be done anytime during the day when the sun is shining, however, in the study I quoted earlier, women's ovulation was helped by morning sunlight). Remove your shoes if weather permits and make contact with the earth whenever possible.

11:00-12:00pm

Meditation/visualization (after looking at my vision board) and "Fertility Bodywork" routine for increased circulation. (Most of the massages should not be done during your period or if you think you may have conceived).

12:00-1:00pm

Eat Lunch (possibilities include: fertility salad with soy nuts, fertility yogurt, bean soup, salmon salad sandwich on whole wheat or soy bread, peanut/almond butter sandwich on whole wheat or soy bread, sliced avocado sandwich with tomatoes and lettuce on whole grain or soy bread, egg salad sandwich on wheat or soy bread (made with DHA fortified eggs) guacamole with salsa and whole grain chips, a serving of my home made juiced vegetables and a piece of fruit from my fertility diet list)

Take 2 tablespoons flax meal (ground flax seeds) or this can be done at the evening meal or snack

Take supplements as recommended previously in my pregnancy protocol: i.e. multivitamin with vitamin E, folic acid, fish oils, etc. Most supplements are best taken with meals, you can split them between lunch and dinner.

1-3:30pm

Work
My part time teaching schedule varied, but I frequently worked in the afternoons. My biggest suggestion about work and career is if you must work, keep stress levels at a minimum. Be sure to wear loose stretchable clothing which helps with pelvic circulation and flat shoes (high heels throw the body out of alignment). Pack your lunch with some of the more "portable" choices like the sandwiches in my recipe section and bring your own beverage like the fertility tea. If you can, during lunch or breaks, take a walk outside without shoes (if possible) and/or without sun glasses if the sun is shining. If your employer is open to the idea, sit on a "fit ball" to help your

posture and keep circulation in your pelvic area. This is recommended in my "Fertility Bodywork" video.

3:30-4:00pm

Snack: Eat one or two servings of greens (already prepared) and a can of vegetable juice (other options include a green smoothie or a serving of my homemade juiced vegetables) and/or a piece of fruit.

4:00-4:30pm

Meditation and visualization (or this second meditation can be done in the evening).

5:30-6:30pm

Dinner (I would prepare a normal dinner with my husband but I would be sure to add another 2 servings of hormone regulating vegetables.) If my husband was not home for dinner, I would eat from my fertility diet menu.

Take other half of supplements

6:30-10pm

During this time, I would be sure to do the following:
- Use castor oil pack as recommended in the chapter on Fertility Bodywork, then take another ice/hot bath (only the first part of my cycle).
- If I was on the second half of my cycle I would use natural progesterone cream.
- Attend my infertility support group on its designated evening
- Relax before bed, if watching TV, I would watch uplifting or funny programs, especially funny videos

Putting It All Together

- Depending on cycle day, have intercourse on days 11, 13, 15 (keeping feet raised for 15 minute after). Remember, your cycle days may vary depending on your ovulation pattern.
- Take a baby aspirin (remember to check with your doctor)
- Go to bed by 10:30-11:00pm with black-out shades on the window

Chapter 11
Just For Men

Most of this book is written for women in their late 30's and 40's who want to get pregnant naturally. However, as we all know, there is another piece of the equation. A high percentage of couples experience male factor infertility. There is much men can do to enhance their fertility naturally. As I previously mentioned, we did not have a problem with my husband's sperm count, however, you should have your own sperm count tested just to see if your sperm count is too low for fertilization and conception. Even if your sperm count is normal, it just makes sense that if you're trying to conceive, both of you should be doing all you can to optimize your probability of success. Many women experiencing miscarriage or recurrent miscarriage actually may have a problem with their partner's sperm. Some cases of unexplained miscarriage can be traced back to sperm defects even if the count and mobility are normal. This section includes my research on enhancing male fertility.

Anatomical Abnormalities

There are a number of physical abnormalities which can affect men's fertility such as varicoceles (enlarged veins in the scrotum) and undescended testicles just to name a few. If you are having trouble conceiving, of course, talk to your doctor or urologist to rule out physical abnormalities which could be affecting your sperm count.

Body Weight and Sperm Quality/Quantity

Obese men have a worse sperm analysis than men whose weight is in the normal range, "there is emerging evidence that male obesity negatively impacts fertility through changes to hormone levels, as well as direct changes to sperm function and sperm molecular composition.[98] There may even be risks for men who are even slightly overweight. To calculate your Body Mass Index (BMI), see my "Pregnancy Protocol" chapter. I should also mention here that when both the man and woman have a BMI which is too low or too high, that could spell double trouble when trying to conceive.

High Blood Pressure

Aside from high blood pressure being an underlying cause of premature death among men and women, men are more likely to have erectile dysfunction if they have high blood pressure.[99] Both the hypertension itself and the medications can be problematic. Many times, high blood pressure can be controlled with a combination of weight loss, diet and exercise. If you do need to go on antihypertensive medication, make sure you talk with your doctor about prescribing a drug which will not cause erectile dysfunction or affect your sperm count or sperm quality.

---

[98] Nicole O. Palmer, Hassan W. Bakos, Tod Fullston, Michelle Lane, Impact of obesity on male fertility, sperm function and molecular composition, Spermatogenesis Vol. 2, Iss. 4, 2012

[99] The Link Between High Blood Pressure Medication, Hypertension, and ED. (n.d.). Retrieved March 30, 2015, from http://www.healthline.com/health/high-blood-pressure-hypertension-linked-to-erectile-dysfunction

Stress

Much has been written about how stress can affect women's fertility, but stress can also affect men's fertility. Stressful life events and perceived stress in men were shown to affect motility and morphology of sperm.[100]

Sleep

One study showed that men who had sleep disturbances or got less than 6 hours of sleep per night had lower sperm concentration, sperm count, motility and quality.[101]

Exercise

Some exercise is good for fertility, and likewise, a sedentary lifestyle can reduce sperm count. One study found that men who watched more than 20 hours of TV weekly had a 44% lower sperm count than those who watched almost no TV. Men who exercised for 15 or more hours weekly at a moderate to vigorous rate had a 73% higher sperm count than those who exercised less than 5 hours per week.[102]

Intercourse

I conceived four times by having intercourse on days 11, 13, and 15 of my cycle. As I mentioned earlier, there is

---

[100] Janevic, Teresa et al., Effects of work and life stress on semen quality Fertility and Sterility, Volume 102, Issue 2, 530 - 538

[101] Tina Kold Jensen, Anna-Maria Andersson, Niels Erik Skakkebæk, Ulla Nordstrøm Joensen, Martin Blomberg Jensen, Tina Harmer Lassen, Loa Nordkap, Inge Alhmann Olesen, Åse Marie Hansen, Naja Hulvej Rod, and Niels Jørgensen, Association of Sleep Disturbances With Reduced Semen Quality: A Cross-sectional Study Among 953 Healthy Young Danish Men Am. J. Epidemiol. (2013) 177 (10): 1027-1037 first published online April 7, 2013 doi:10.1093/aje/kws420

[102] Datz, T. (n.d.). TV viewing, exercise habits may significantly affect sperm count. Retrieved March 30, 2014, from http://www.hsph.harvard.edu/news/press-releases/tv-viewing-exercise-habits-may-significantly-affect-sperm-count/

conflicting information about whether or not daily intercourse is better than having intercourse every 48 hours. Having intercourse every other day is thought to replenish the sperm supply. On the other hand, one Australian researcher found that men who ejaculated daily had a 12% drop in sperm DNA damage. The theory is the longer sperm are in the testes, the more likely they are to accumulate DNA damage and the warm environment could make them slower. But frequent ejaculation also decreased semen volume and sperm concentrations but it did not compromise sperm motility and, in fact, this rose slightly but significantly.[103]

As mentioned earlier, we were able to conceive multiple times having intercourse every other day even with one fallopian tube. Daily intercourse would have been too demanding for us. In any event, be sure to start having intercourse on day 11 (again, you need to adjust this for your cycle as discussed in my section on timing intercourse) because you want to make sure that the sperm has time to travel up into the fallopian tube *before* ovulation.

Lubricants

Most vaginal lubricants are harmful to sperm. However there are a few on the market that are not. Look for lubricants that are sperm friendly if you absolutely need a vaginal lubricant during intercourse. Some sources actually recommend using egg whites if you need lubrication. If at all possible, do not lubricants.

---

[103] European Society of Human Reproduction and Embryology (ESHRE). (2009, July 1). Daily Sex Helps Reduce Sperm DNA Damage And Improve Fertility. ScienceDaily. Retrieved May 8, 2015 from www.sciencedaily.com/releases/2009/06/090630075311.htm

Medications

Certain medications can interfere with sperm production. Some of these include cimetidine (an acid reducer), some blood pressure medications, certain antibiotics, some medications taken for depression including SSRI's, some arthritis medications and cancer chemotherapy drugs. If you are suffering from erectile dysfunction, one of the popular ED drugs has been associated with sperm damage. Talk with your doctor if you need to take medications for any reason to find out if the drug you are taking affects sperm production or quality. If it does, there may be alternatives.

Hot Showers, Saunas, Hot Tubs

Try to avoid long hot showers, saunas, baths, hot tubs, etc. The testes are normally cooler than the rest of the body and this is important for sperm production. A number of studies have confirmed that a rise in scrotal temperature will temporarily reduce sperm count.

Laptop Computers

Using laptop computers may also raise scrotal temperature. Part of the increase in temperature is attributed to the heat generated by the computer itself and another part of the increase is attributed to the position men must sit in to balance a computer on their lap (with their thighs close together). If you do use a laptop computer, sit at a desk. Do not put the computer directly on your lap. Also, one study done on men using wireless internet-connected laptops for 4 hours showed a significant decrease in progressive sperm motility and an increase in sperm DNA fragmentation.[104]

Boxers vs. Briefs?

There actually is no evidence that wearing boxers vs. briefs is better for male fertility. Most people think that briefs will warm the testicles more because they're tighter and worn closer to the body. Maybe that's true, but it hasn't been proven to lower fertility. You be the judge, if you want to try boxers, there's no harm in it.

Oral Hygiene

What could seeing your dentist possibly have to do with fertility? Oral bacteria can infect the reproductive system causing "bacteriospermia" or an infection of the semen. A statistically significant association was found between poor oral hygiene and subnormal sperm count across all age groups.[105] It's a good idea to see your dentist and have your teeth cleaned regularly.

Diet and Supplements To Enhance Male Fertility

The following supplements have been found to be fertility boosters in men:

---

[104] Avendaño, Conrado et al., Use of laptop computers connected to internet through Wi-Fi decreases human sperm motility and increases sperm DNA fragmentation, Fertility and Sterility, Volume 97, Issue 1, 39 - 45.e2

[105] Nwhator SO, Umeizudike KA, Ayanbadejo PO, Opeodu OI, Olamijulo JA, Sorsa T, Another reason for impeccable oral hygiene: oral hygiene-sperm count link, J Contemp Dent Pract. 2014 May 1;15(3):352-8.

Zinc and Folic Acid

Zinc and Folic acid taken together have shown to increase the sperm count in subfertile and fertile men.[106] Folic Acid may be found in green leafy vegetables, legumes, oranges and fortified cereals. Zinc is found in red meat, poultry, and fortified cereals. You may want to take a supplement if you can't get these through your diet.

Selenium, Vitamin E

Selenium taken with vitamin E improves sperm motility according to one study.[107] Selenium may prevent sperm damage and is found in seafood, meat, liver, and grains and Brazil nuts. It is usually present in multivitamins. Vitamin E may also be taken as a supplement (the men in the study were given 400 IU daily).

Omega-3 Fatty Acids

Earlier, I spoke about prostaglandins for female fertility. Sperm have naturally occurring prostaglandins as well. Men should do everything they can to manufacture the "good" prostaglandins which will help with sperm quality. Some men with poorly functioning sperm have been found to have low levels of the good prostaglandins. You should be eating a diet rich in Omega-3 fatty acids. Studies have confirmed that men with a diet rich in EPA and DHA had an improvement in semen quality.[108] See my fertility diet

---

[106] Wong WY, Merkus HM, Thomas CM, Menkveld R, Zielhuis GA, Steegers-Theunissen RP, Effects of folic acid and zinc sulfate on male factor subfertility: a double-blind, randomized, placebo-controlled trial, Fertil Steril. 2002 Mar;77(3):491-8

[107] Moslemi, M. K., & Tavanbakhsh, S. (2011). Selenium–vitamin E supplementation in infertile men: effects on semen parameters and pregnancy rate. International Journal of General Medicine, 4, 99–104. doi:10.2147/IJGM.S16275

[108] Safarinejad MR, Effect of omega-3 polyunsaturated fatty acid supplementation on semen profile and enzymatic anti-oxidant capacity of seminal plasma in infertile men with idiopathic oligoasthenoteratospermia: a double-blind, placebo-controlled,

section for food sources. You could also consider taking a supplement.

L-Arginine, L-Carnitine, Acetyl Carnitine

L-Arginine can help with the quality and quantity of sperm. It is an amino acid which is found in the head of the sperm. L-Carnitine is an amino acid which helps with the motility and volume of sperm. It also helps with the formation (size and shape) and proper maturation of sperm. One study examined the effect of treatment with carnitine, acetyl carnitine, L-arginine (along with ginseng). These had a significant improvement in progressive sperm motility.[109]

Vitamin D

As I mentioned in my fertility supplements one study found vitamin D can help with sperm quality and testosterone production.[110]

Vitamin C

Vitamin C has been shown to enhance sperm quality by protecting it from DNA damage. If the sperm's DNA is damaged, and conception occurs, it could lead to miscarriage, or possibly chromosomal damage and birth defects. Vitamin C improves sperm count, sperm motility, and sperm morphology.[111] In an analysis of 80 healthy

---

randomised study, Andrologia. 2011 Feb;43(1):38-47. doi: 10.1111/j.1439-0272.2009.01013.x. Epub 2010 Dec 19.

[109] Morgante G, Scolaro V, Tosti C, Di Sabatino A, Piomboni P, De Leo V, Treatment with carnitine, acetyl carnitine, L-arginine and ginseng improves sperm motility and sexual health in men with asthenopermia, Minerva Urol Nefrol. 2010 Sep;62(3):213-8.

[110] Elisabeth Lerchbaum, and Barbara R Obermayer-Pietsch, Vitamin D and fertility-a systematic review, Eur J Endocrinol January 24, 2012 EJE-11-0984

[111] Akmal M, Qadri JQ, Al-Waili NS, Thangal S, Haq A, Saloom KY, Improvement in human semen quality after oral supplementation of vitamin C, J Med Food. 2006 Fall;9(3):440-2.

male volunteers between 22 and 80 years of age, the scientists found that men older than 44 who consumed the most vitamin C had 20 percent less sperm DNA damage compared to men older than 44 who consumed the least vitamin C. The same was true for vitamin E, zinc, and folate.[112]

Coffee/Caffeine

Whether or not coffee or caffeine is good or bad for your health seems to keep changing. However, even though coffee and caffeine aren't good for women trying to conceive, coffee may help sperm motility in lower amounts and hurt sperm in higher amounts. One study found: "in doses of 3 and 6 mm/ml, caffeine significantly increased the percentage of motile sperm, but it had no influence on sperm velocity. In doses greater than 6 mm/ml, caffeine exhibited a slight insignificant stimulation that reversed later into an inhibitory effect on all parameters of sperm motility in a dose of 60 mm/ml. Reaching a dose of 120 mm/ml, caffeine caused complete immobilization of human spermatozoa."[113] Since it's almost impossible to measure how much caffeine you are consuming, it would be a good idea to cut it out of your diet.

Things to Avoid:

Soy

Although I made soy a regular part of my diet when I was trying to conceive, there is evidence that the plant estrogens in soy could have a negative effect on sperm production. One study found that "higher intake of soy foods and soy

---

[112] Schmid, Thomas E. et al.,Micronutrients intake is associated with improved sperm DNA quality in older men, Fertility and Sterility, Volume 98, Issue 5, 1130 - 1137.e1

[113] Moussa MM, Caffeine and sperm motility, Fertil Steril. 1983 Jun;39(6):845-8.

isoflavones is associated with lower sperm concentration."[114]

Xenoestrogens

I previously spoke about and listed sources of xenoestrogens (environmental toxins which may mimic estrogen). Men should also avoid xenoestrogens as these may have an effect on hormones and sperm production.

Alcohol

I've already mentioned that women who are trying to conceive should avoid alcohol consumption, but men whose partners are trying to conceive should avoid it as well. There is a higher rate of miscarriage in women who had partners who drank around the time of conception (about 10 drinks per week).[115] If you're trying to conceive, cut the alcohol out of your diet, or reduce it significantly.

Marijuana

Smoking marijuana has been shown to reduce seminal fluid and reduce sperm count. In addition, the sperm of men who smoke Marijuana seem to swim abnormally and have a harder time attaching to the egg before fertilization.[116]

---

[114] Jorge E. Chavarro, Thomas L. Toth, Sonita M. Sadio, and Russ Hauser. Soy food and isoflavone intake in relation to semen quality parameters among men from an infertility clinic. Human Reproduction, July 24, 2008 DOI: 10.1093/humrep/den243

[115] Tine Brink Henriksen, Niels Henrik Hjollund, Tina Kold Jensen, Jens Peter Bonde, Anna-Maria Andersson, Henrik Kolstad, Erik Ernst, Aleksander Giwercman, Niels Erik Skakkebæk Jørn Olsen,Alcohol Consumption at the Time of Conception and Spontaneous Abortion, Am. J. Epidemiol. (2004) 160 (7): 661-667. doi: 10.1093/aje/kwh259

[116] Nordqvist, C. (2003, October 14). "Marijuana smoking may damage sperm." Medical News Today. Retrieved from, http://www.medicalnewstoday.com/articles/4482.php.

Cigarettes

Of course, you already know the dangers of smoking. But if you're trying to conceive, smoking can impair your sperm's ability to fertilize an egg. Smokers were found to possess significantly decreased density (number) and motility of their sperm than nonsmokers.[117] In addition, smoking can lead to erectile dysfunction because it affects male sex hormones. Worst of all, if you do succeed in getting pregnant, smoking could damage your DNA which could be passed on to your baby.

Cell Phones

It is possible that radiation from cell phones might negatively affect a man's sperm especially when kept in their pant pockets. This may be true even if your cell phone is on and you're not talking. In control groups, 50-85% of sperm have normal movement. The researchers in one study found this proportion fell by an average of 8 percentage points when there was exposure to mobile phones. Similar effects were seen for sperm viability.[118] It may be a good idea to turn your cell phone off when you're not using it.

Car Exhaust and Traffic Fumes

It is thought that men exposed to traffic fumes every day suffer a reduction in the quality of their sperm.

---

[117] Kulikauskas V, Blaustein D, Ablin RJ., Cigarette smoking and its possible effects on sperm.,Fertil Steril. 1985 Oct;44(4):526-8.
[118] Mobile phones negatively affect male fertility, new study suggests. (2014, May 10). Retrieved March 30, 2015, from http://www.exeter.ac.uk/news/featurednews/title_385859_en.html

Toxic Chemicals

Here are some chemicals to avoid to the greatest degree possible:

- Alkylating agents (used in drug manufacturing and chemotherapy)
- Nitrous Oxide and anesthetic Agents
- Metals such as lead, mercury, cadmium, & boron
- Carbon tetrachloride (used in dry cleaning)
- Chloroprene – (used in rubber manufacturing)
- Ethylene Oxide (used to sterilize)
- Tris (flame retardant used in the clothing industry)
- Pesticides such as dibromochlorpropane, ethylene dibromide, chlordecone, and chlordane (even low levels of pesticides found in foods could be harmful so eat organic foods if possible)
- Solvents such as carbon disulfide and glycol ethers
- Vinyl chloride - Vinyl chloride is used to make PVC. PVC is used to make some plastic products.

There are many other workplace chemicals that could be hazardous. Employers are required to keep MSDS's (Material Safety Data Sheets) which, by law, employers should make available. These data sheets have information on the workplace chemicals which employees may be exposed to on the job. If you are concerned about your work environment, ask your employer if you can view these data sheets. You may also get more information on hazardous workplace chemicals from the OSHA (Occupational Safety and Health Administration) website: www.OSHA.gov.

If you work around chemicals, it's best to be in a well ventilated area. Do not eat or drink within close proximity of toxic substances. Avoid skin contact with chemicals. Ask your employer for protective equipment such as gloves, masks, etc.

Chapter 12
Preventing and Dealing with Miscarriage

I firmly believe that preventing miscarriage, starts in whole or in part, by what you do *before* you get pregnant. As I've mentioned throughout this book, hormonal balance and overall health help to create the optimal environment for conception and pregnancy. This chapter may reiterate points I've already mentioned in the book elsewhere and it contains other research I've found on preventing miscarriage.

Trying To Get Pregnant Again After a Miscarriage

It used to be recommended to wait before trying to get pregnant after a miscarriage. However, recent research has shown that there is no need to wait to conceive again. In one study, researchers found that women who got pregnant again within six months were actually less likely to miscarry again.[119] If you carried a baby near term (perhaps with a stillbirth), or if you had a D&C you will be told to wait before trying again and of course you should follow your doctor's advice.

If you've had a miscarriage, give yourself time to grieve. I had a memorial service for each pregnancy I lost. This was

---

[119] Julie DaVanzo1, Lauren Hale, Mizanur Rahman, How long after a miscarriage should women wait before becoming pregnant again? Multivariate analysis of cohort data from Matlab, Bangladesh, BMJ Open 2012;2:e001591 doi:10.1136/bmjopen-2012-001591

alone, in private, but it helped to acknowledge that I a baby. It wasn't just an embryo or a cluster of cells. This was my child. I know, for me, there initially was a feeling like I had to start trying to get pregnant again immediately (especially since I was in my 40's), but I came to the realization that since I had to wait before trying to conceive again anyway (at least with my ectopic pregnancy and the miscarriages that required a D&C), I needed to use that time to acknowledge my pain, feel it, and move on. It really is a relief to just get mad, to not be strong, and to fall apart - even if for just a short time.

Recurrent miscarriage can be overcome. Even though the doctors labeled me a "habitual aborter" (the medical term for recurrent miscarriage - which I find quite offensive), I was able to regain control of my body and have a perfectly normal pregnancy without medical intervention – even after six miscarriages. This proved to me that I am in control of life. I can create my own reality. Even under the worst of circumstances, I had to pick myself up and know that when the time is right, things will fall into place. Don't think you'll never get pregnant again or carry a pregnancy to term. Miscarriage is a common occurrence. Most women who've had one go on to have one or more children. As I mentioned earlier, once you've moved through the pain and disappointment, dare to dream again. Don't fall into the trap of saying "I'm not getting my hopes up again, only to be disappointed."

Are you more fertile after a miscarriage?

There are many so called old wives tales that claim it's easier to get pregnant after a miscarriage (probably because of increased progesterone levels). Is it true? Well there may be some evidence that you are more fertile after pregnancy loss, but the research is limited. One study conducted at the Boston University School of Medicine found a positive relationship between early pregnancy loss and subsequent fertility.[120]

Ectopic Pregnancy and Getting Pregnant Again

One of the most devastating experiences I went through was having an ectopic pregnancy. If you are trying to get pregnant naturally, you feel like the removal of one of your fallopian tubes is a major setback because it can essentially cut your chances of conceiving in half. Aside from the inevitable depression that follows most miscarriages, you may be feeling the time pressure because of your age. As long as you still have one tube, you can still get pregnant. And, even though I was over the age of 40, I conceived 4 times with only one fallopian tube. So, optimally it would great to have both tubes, but you can still do just fine with one. According to a study published in Human Reproduction, your chances of getting pregnant after an ectopic may be as high as 70%.[121] Interestingly, my mother's first pregnancy was ectopic and she went on to have three children. Tubal pregnancies require immediate attention and frequently require surgery to remove the fallopian tube. Sometimes, a drug called methotrexate (which I received for my second ectopic) can be given if the tubal pregnancy is caught early enough. This drug will stop the growth of the pregnancy and help it to expel naturally. This may preserve the affected tube.

When I was going through fertility treatments, my doctor told me I had to wait until I had 3 full menstrual cycles

---

[120] Wang X[1], Chen C, Wang L, Chen D, Guang W, French J.
Fertil Steril. 2003 Mar;79(3):577-84. Conception, early pregnancy loss, and time to clinical pregnancy: a population-based prospective study
[121] Hervé Fernandez, Perrine Capmas, Jean Philippe Lucot, Benoit Resch, Pierre Panel, and Jean Bouyer for the GROG Fertility after ectopic pregnancy: the DEMETER randomized trial Hum. Reprod. 2013 : det037v1-det037.

after my ectopic before we could try again. *What??? Three Months???* That sounded like an eternity. Even if your ectopic pregnancy is treated medically with methotrexate, you are warned not to conceive for a full three months after being given this drug because it could cause birth defects if you conceive while it is in your system.

Causes of Miscarriage & Possible Prevention

Chromosomal Abnormalities

When women over 40 have miscarriages, I think it's very tempting for the medical community to blame it on chromosomal abnormalities because your eggs are older and it's possible that many of the "good" eggs already ovulated when you were younger. Nobody knows for sure why I miscarried so many times (except for the ectopic pregnancies), but I didn't buy the "old eggs" explanation. Yes, it is true that older women have had their eggs inside of them longer and the eggs may have been exposed to more toxins, environmental radiation, and just the normal wear and tear associated with the aging process, but unless you have genetic testing on the fetal tissue, there is no way to know for sure if your miscarriage was caused as a result of a chromosomal error.

Women of all ages may experience miscarriage as a result of a chromosomal abnormality, it's not just a problem in older women. I would constantly tell myself, "There's a good egg in there somewhere, I'm going to be good and ready when it shows up!"

Stress and Miscarriage

The scientific community is hesitant to draw a clear cut link between stress and miscarriage, however, some studies have shown that there is an increased risk of miscarriage in women who are under high levels of stress both before conception and in early pregnancy. When under physical or emotional stress, stress hormones are secreted which can lead to uterine contractions. Stress hormones cause a chain reaction which can negatively affect the development of the embryo and the placenta. Even more convincing is that these stress hormones have actually been found in the tissue of fetuses of women who experienced recurrent miscarriage. A study done at Tufts University School of Medicine found that stress and stress related hormones and chemicals produce physiologic changes and reactions in the uterus. Women in the study who experienced one or more miscarriages had high levels of these chemicals which are thought to destroy tissue and disrupt the placenta.[122]

Weight and Miscarriage

There does seem to be some evidence that women who are underweight before they become pregnant may be more likely to miscarry. Likewise, women who are obese are also more likely to miscarry even if they don't suffer from diabetes. One study found "underweight and obese women are at a higher risk of miscarriage than women with normal weight. Reproductive potential in obese women is decreased as a result of impaired folliculogenesis, ovulation and conception, and obesity is associated with an increased risk of pregnancy complications. In spontaneous pregnancies, obesity has been found to be an independent cause of miscarriage. A low body mass may also be a risk factor for menstrual disturbances and infertility problems. Recently, women with a pre-pregnant BMI < 18.5 kg/m^2

---

[122] J Clin Endocrinol Metab. 2003 Nov;88(11):5580; author reply 5580-1.High levels of intrauterine corticotrophin-releasing hormone, urocortin, tryptase, and interleukin-8 in spontaneous abortions.
Florio P, Ciarmela P, Arcuri F, Petraglia F.

have been found to have 1.7-fold increased risk of miscarriage in spontaneous pregnancies."[123] As mentioned before, it is extremely important to deal with your weight issues before trying to conceive.

Depression and Miscarriage

Does miscarriage cause depression, or does depression cause miscarriage? Well...maybe both. Studies have shown a higher rate of miscarriage in depressed women.[124] If you are currently on antidepressant medication or if your doctor recommends medication for your depression, you should discuss your plans to get pregnant and how your medications will affect your pregnancy. One study showed a higher rate of pre-eclampsia in women on anti-depressants.[125] Treatment doesn't always involve medication. It may be helpful just to talk to a professional or review my chapter on how I became my own therapist. It really did help.

The depression and anxiety experienced by many women after a miscarriage can continue for years, even after the birth of a healthy child. According to a study published online by the *British Journal of Psychiatry*:

---

[123] Zdravka Veleva,Aila Tiitinen,Sirpa Vilska,Christel Hydén-Granskog,Candido Tomás,Hannu Martikainen,and Juha S. Tapanainen
High and low BMI increase the risk of miscarriage after IVF/ICSI and FET Hum. Reprod. (2008) 23 (4): 878-884 first published online February 15, 2008 doi:10.1093/humrep/den017

[124] Mayumi Sugiura-Ogasawara, Toshiaki A. Furukawa, Yumi Nakano, Shiro Hori, Koji Aoki, and Toshinori Kitamura, Depression as a potential causal factor in subsequent miscarriage in recurrent spontaneous aborters Hum. Reprod. (2002) 17 (10): 2580-2584 doi:10.1093/humrep/17.10.2580

[125] Kristin Palmsten, Soko Setoguchi, Andrea V. Margulis, Amanda R. Patrick and Sonia Hernández-Díaz, Elevated Risk of Preeclampsia in Pregnant Women With Depression: Depression or Antidepressants?, Am. J. Epidemiol. (2012) doi: 10.1093/aje/kwr394 First published online: March 22, 2012

"Depression and anxiety associated with a previous prenatal loss shows a persisting pattern that continues after the birth of a subsequent (healthy) child. Interventions targeting women with previous prenatal loss may improve the health outcomes of women and their children."
"Given the adverse outcomes of persistent maternal depression on both child and family outcomes, early recognition of symptoms can lead to preventive interventions to reduce the burden of illness, provide coping strategies to reduce anxiety and depression and promote healthy adjustment of the mother, family and child."[126]

In my case, I do think I experienced some depression after my miscarriages (especially the first two) although I never received a clinical diagnosis. I don't think I had long lasting effects of depression, but I will say that all through my pregnancy and even after my daughter was born, I had irrational fears that she was going to die either in utero or from SIDS after birth. Even now that she is older, I tend to catch myself worrying about all the possible things that could harm her. You just can't go through that much loss without some type of psychological trauma.

Intercourse Mistiming

Earlier, when I discussed my pregnancy protocol, I recommended having intercourse on days 11, 13, and 15 because ovulation can be somewhat unpredictable. Even though some sources say to have intercourse within 48 hours of ovulation, if you wait too long to have intercourse after ovulation, and the egg should fertilize, it may be prone

---

[126] Previous prenatal loss as a predictor of perinatal depression and anxiety
Emma Robertson Blackmore, Denise Côté-Arsenault, Wan Tang, Vivette Glover, Jonathan Evans, Jean Golding, Thomas G. O'Connor
DOI: 10.1192/bjp.bp.110.083105 Published 27 April 2011

to miscarriage since it may have started to deteriorate. It's best to have the sperm ready and waiting *before* a woman ovulates. There may be reason to believe that a woman's most fertile time actually ends on the day of ovulation because an egg can start breaking down as soon as the day after (see my pregnancy protocol chapter on timing intercourse).

D&C

I had a number of D&C's after my miscarriages and it always worried me to be having yet another surgery. I really didn't want more surgical instruments poking around inside of me. If you've ever seen the instrument they use for a D&C, it's pretty scary looking. In general, most early miscarriages will expel naturally. However, many women opt for surgical removal because it gets it over with quickly and it usually puts an end to your pregnancy symptoms. After one of my miscarriages, my hCG levels kept going up and up, and finally my doctor strongly suggested a D&C because he thought it might be a molar pregnancy (which is when the cells keep dividing and may turn malignant). Well, it turns out it wasn't a molar pregnancy, but my doctor did have a hard time getting the bleeding to stop after the procedure.

A D&C is usually done as an outpatient in a hospital or other surgical center. You should be given some light anesthesia (once I was given IV Valium which worked fine). Ahead of time, they may insert something called a Laminaria stick (which is a seaweed stick) to help dilate your cervix. This stick absorbs water and grows which should expand your cervix when in place. You will be placed on a gynecological type examining table with your feet in stirrups. The doctor will use an instrument called a "curette" which is metal and has a curved shaped loop. The walls of the uterus are scraped to remove what remains of the pregnancy so it may expel. This may also be called a surgical evacuation of the uterus or a D&E.

The risks include: infection, bleeding, scarring & adhesions, and even perforation of the uterus and other organs. Although these complications are rare, some of them could harm your future fertility. You may also have to wait longer after a D&C to try to conceive again because your uterus needs to heal and the endometrial lining needs to build back up.

Infection

A common bacterial infection of the vagina (bacterial vaginosis) has shown to double the rate of miscarriage in the first three months of pregnancy and increase the risk of premature birth.[127] A common symptom of this condition is an abnormal vaginal discharge. There are other infections of the reproductive system that have been associated with infertility and miscarriage. Sometimes women with these infections have no symptoms at all, however, antibiotic therapy may be all they need to conceive and carry to term. These infections should be treated *before* you try to conceive – you do not want to be taking antibiotics while you are pregnant. Talk with your doctor if you think you might have an infection or ask if you can be tested.

---

[127] Deborah B. Nelson, George Macones, Bacterial Vaginosis in Pregnancy: Current Findings and Future Directions, Epidemiol Rev (2002) 24 (2): 102-108. doi: 10.1093/epirev/mxf008

Progesterone Deficiency

Progesterone deficiency could result in miscarriage. When a woman becomes pregnant, the corpus luteum produces progesterone which helps to support the pregnancy. The corpus luteum is formed from the ovarian follicle after the egg is released at the time of ovulation. If pregnancy occurs, after about 9-10 weeks, the placenta should take over progesterone production. If the corpus luteum doesn't produce enough progesterone initially, it could result in an early pregnancy loss. I should say that the effectiveness of progesterone supplementation seems to be inconclusive. I've read some studies that showed higher success rates when women's pregnancies were supported with progesterone. I asked one of my doctors about giving me progesterone (when I was trying to conceive naturally) and he was absolutely against it (I still wonder if I should have sought a second opinion). My best advice is to talk with your doctor about whether or not it might be right for you. I did use natural progesterone cream while I was trying to conceive, but I did not continue it once I found out I was pregnant. It is possible that this cream may have helped support my pregnancy initially, but there's no way to know for sure.

Celiac Disease, Infertility, Miscarriage, and Fetal Growth Retardation

Celiac disease is also known as gluten intolerance (gluten is usually found in wheat, rye and barley). Basically, celiac disease can create an inability of the intestine to absorb certain nutrients from food. Symptoms of celiac disease may be weight loss, rash, joint pain, mouth sores, muscle cramps, diarrhea, gas, bloating, and the list goes on. As far as fertility and miscarriage, one recent study associated celiac disease with significant increases in spontaneous abortion, premature delivery, and later age of menarche.[128] If you think you may have celiac disease, talk with your doctor about possible testing. You may benefit from a gluten free diet.

Electric and Magnetic Fields (EMF's)

Electric and magnetic fields come from power lines, appliances, electrical wiring, equipment, computers among other things. A number of studies have been done on the effects of prolonged exposure to high electric and magnetic fields. I should say that there is conflicting information about the hazard EMF's pose to pregnant women. In terms of fertility and miscarriage, some sources claim that there is an increased incidence of infertility, miscarriage, birth defects and even some cancers in babies when the mother was exposed to high EMF's. Almost anything that is plugged in gives off an electric field. To give off a magnetic field, the item must be plugged in and operating. There is quite a bit of variability in the EMF's given off from different appliances or electronic devices. Here are some things to avoid to the greatest degree possible:
- Electric heating pads, humidifiers, heated waterbeds
- Prolonged computer use (about 20 or more hrs. per week)
- Electric blankets have been associated with a higher miscarriage rate.
- Don't sit too close to the television, microwave or other electronic devices when in use as the further away you are from an appliance or electronic device, the less exposure you will have to it's EMF (although some EMF's can penetrate through walls.)

---

[128] Stephanie M. Moleski, Christina C. Lindenmeyer, J. Jon Veloski, Robin S. Miller, Cynthia L. Miller, David Kastenberg, Anthony J. DiMarino, Increased rates of pregnancy complications in women with celiac disease, Ann Gastroenterol 2015; 28 (2): 236-240

- Limit use of wireless devices like smartphones (and wireless landline phones) and tablets – these are thought to have a negative effect on the fetus. Try to keep them away from your belly when using them.

Hot Tubs and Saunas

You should avoid anything that is going to raise your body temperature such as hot tubs and saunas. Raising your core body temperature could increase your risk of miscarriage. Baths and Showers are usually not a problem because your entire body is not immersed and bath water tends to cool over time. If you feel like you're starting to "overheat" get out of the tub as soon as possible.

Nitrates

Avoid nitrates and nitrites which can be harmful to the fetus and possibly increase the risk of miscarriage. Although the research done in this area has found it hard to isolate actual exposure and therefore a cause and effect relationship, it would be a good idea to avoid these substances as much as possible. These compounds are found in processed meats like lunch meats, smoked meats, hot dogs, bacon and many others (read the labels). Well water might also be another source of nitrites. See my pregnancy protocol chapter for information on bottled vs. tap water.

Nutrition

Many miscarriages can be prevented with a diet high in fruits and vegetables and vitamin supplements.[129] It's possible that a diet high in antioxidants can help regulate blood flow

---

[129] Maconochie N, Doyle P, Prior S, Simmons R., Risk factors for first trimester miscarriage--results from a UK-population-based case-control study. BJOG. 2007 Feb;114(2):170-86.

to the placenta avoiding sudden changes which can cause tissue damage. If you are following my fertility diet and taking the recommended supplements, you should be getting a high level of antioxidants.

Dehydration

Dehydration can cause pre-term labor. Be sure to drink plenty of water when you're pregnant. Some women have trouble eating and drinking because of the nausea and vomiting with morning sickness. I found it helpful to heat my drinking water during the first three months of my pregnancy. The warmer water seemed to be easier on my stomach (I had fairly severe nausea with my successful pregnancy).

Coffee/Caffeine

Some studies have shown that women who drank 2-3 cups of coffee per day were found to have a higher risk of miscarriage. Even one daily cup of caffeinated coffee carries a risk – especially since the serving sizes have grown significantly in many fast food coffee shops. Caffeine easily crosses the placenta and may affect cell development.[130] Even though I have historically been a coffee drinker, when I was pregnant, it was repulsive to me.

Medications

Just because a medication is sold over the counter, it doesn't mean it's safe to take during pregnancy. You shouldn't take *anything* before talking with a doctor first. There may be reasons why you need to take medication

---

[130] Xiaoping Weng, Roxana Odouli, De-Kun Li. Maternal caffeine consumption during pregnancy and the risk of miscarriage: a prospective cohort study. American Journal of Obstetrics & Gynecology, 2008; 198 (3): 279.e1-279.e8 DOI: 10.1016/j.ajog.2007.10.803

during pregnancy, however, some drugs have been found to increase the risk of miscarriage and birth defects. Most drugs are classified according to whether or not they are safe to take during pregnancy. If you have any doubts about taking a prescribed drug, it may be helpful to talk with a pharmacist or get a second opinion from another physician. I absolutely did not want to take any drugs while I was pregnant.

Exercise

You should always talk with your doctor about the appropriate level of exercise. Some exercise is good during pregnancy as long as your cervix hasn't been found to be weak. Most of the research I've read recommends *moderate* exercise. Try to avoid anything that is going to raise your core temperature or anything that might involve falling or other trauma (such as skiing). As I mentioned earlier, I did very little exercise when I was pregnant mainly out of fear and first trimester nausea. However, I probably could have benefited from getting at least some exercise.

I should also mention here that there does seem to be some conflicting information about whether or not exercise is associated with miscarriage. However, according to one study, women who engage in high impact exercise in early pregnancy (more than 7 hours per week) were three times more likely to miscarry.[131] I actually had a PA in my OB's office say that I could run a marathon after becoming pregnant and it wouldn't make a difference. I don't believe that and I think women should be cautioned to take it easy. It just makes sense that it would be harder for an embryo to

---

[131] Madsen M, Jørgensen T, Jensen M, Juhl M, Olsen J, Andersen P, Nybo Andersen A. Leisure time physical exercise during pregnancy and the risk of miscarriage: a study within the Danish National Birth Cohort. BJOG 2007;114:1419–1426

implant and take hold properly if your body is bouncing around.

Hazardous Chemicals

Earlier, in my pregnancy protocol chapter, I mentioned things to avoid if you're trying to conceive. Here are a few more chemicals that have been found to increase the risk of miscarriage:

- Perchloroethylene (PERC) – used in dry cleaning, typewriter correction fluid and shoe polish
- Toluene – Toluene is used in making paints, paint thinners, fingernail polish, lacquers, adhesives, rubber and in some printing and leather tanning processes.
- Xylene, acetone, trichloroethylene, and other chemical solvents (acetone is sometimes found in nail polish remover)
- Paint thinners, paint strippers, and glycol ethers in paints
- Car exhaust – this is a source of many toxic substances. When I was pregnant, if I had to walk through a parking lot, the smell of car exhaust would automatically make me gag to the point of vomiting. That should be an indication how devastating it is to your system.
- Anesthesia – a higher rate of birth defects was found in nurses who administer or assist with anesthesia.

There are many other workplace chemicals that could be hazardous. As I mentioned in the "Just For Men" chapter, employers are required to keep MSDS's (Material Safety Data Sheets) which, by law, they should make available to employees. These data sheets have information on the workplace chemicals you may be exposed to on the job. If you are concerned about your work environment, ask your employer if you can view these data sheets. You may also get more information on hazardous workplace chemicals from the OSHA (Occupational Safety and Health Administration) website: www.OSHA.gov.

If you are concerned about your work environment, ask if it is possible to transfer to a safer area when you are pregnant or if you are trying to conceive.

Standing, Lifting and Risk of Miscarriage

Some studies have found an increased risk of miscarriage with standing and lifting at work. Other more recent studies have been unable to substantiate a clear connection, but they advise women to limit these activities.[132]

Night Shift and Miscarriage

Recent reports have claimed that night shift workers have a higher miscarriage rate.[133] The reason why is unknown, however, some possibilities include the increased light exposure has an effect on hormone levels. It's also possible night shifts may be more stressful in terms of the type and hours of work.

Does Bedrest Prevent Miscarriage?

There actually is no evidence that bedrest will prevent miscarriage. However, I should say that later in pregnancy, constant standing or heavy exercise could put too much pressure on the cervix especially if your cervix is weak to

---

[132] Bonde, J. P. E., Jørgensen, K. T., Bonzini, M., & Palmer, K. T. (2013). Risk of miscarriage and occupational activity: a systematic review and meta-analysis regarding shift work, working hours, lifting, standing and physical workload. Scandinavian Journal of Work, Environment & Health, 39(4), 325–334. doi:10.5271/sjweh.3337

[133] Fertility experts say night shift workers 'more likely to suffer miscarriages' (2013, July 9). Retrieved March 30, 2015, from:
http://www.uhs.nhs.uk/AboutTheTrust/Newsandpublications/Latestnews/2013/Fertility-experts-say-night-shift-workers-more-likely-to-suffer-miscarriages.aspx

begin with (a condition called cervical incompetence). During my successful pregnancy, I decreased my activity level drastically. Part of this was because I was too scared to do anything, but the other part was that I had read that you shouldn't put too much pressure on your cervix by standing, lifting, etc. I was always worried that I was going to have a premature birth (which I did not), so I did everything I could to prevent it. When you do get pregnant, talk to your doctor about what activity level is best for you.

Does Spotting Mean You're Going To Miscarry?

Spotting isn't necessarily a good sign, but it certainly doesn't mean you're going to miscarry. I've heard estimates as high as 25-30% of all pregnancies have some spotting. This can be cause by a variety of conditions from yeast infections to implantation bleeding. I had spotting with all my pregnancies, including my successful pregnancy. When I was pregnant with my daughter, I spotted for a full three months. It appeared, from the ultrasound, that some implantation blood was trapped between the uterus and the gestational sac. It was coming out very slowly which led to the spotting. I also had a few other incidences of spotting during my successful pregnancy. Although no definitive reason was found, it obviously didn't lead to a miscarriage. One study found that spotting and light episodes of bleeding are not associated with miscarriage, especially if only lasting 1–2 days.[134] If you are pregnant and you are spotting, it's a good idea to see your doctor. Spotting can be an indicator of more severe problems, but having said that, I found the

---

[134] Hasan, R., Baird, D. D., Herring, A. H., Olshan, A. F., Jonsson Funk, M. L., & Hartmann, K. E. (2009). Association Between First-Trimester Vaginal Bleeding and Miscarriage. Obstetrics and Gynecology, 114(4), 860–867. doi:10.1097/AOG.0b013e3181b79796

medical community to be rather unconcerned with most cases of spotting (obviously it's quite common). If nothing else, they can help put your mind at ease.

What supplements can help prevent miscarriage?

Prenatal Vitamins

Prenatal vitamins are specially formulated for pregnant women. Prior to conception, as I mentioned earlier in my pregnancy protocol, I took a multivitamin and some additional supplements. When you do become pregnant, ask your doctor about taking a prenatal vitamin. Here are some important components of multivitamins and/or prenatal vitamins to look for to help prevent miscarriage:

Folic Acid

Folic acid can help prevent some birth defects and women with low folate levels have a higher rate of early miscarriage (as mentioned earlier, folic acid is also especially important to take before you conceive).

Selenium

Women with low selenium levels also have a higher miscarriage rate.[135] Selenium supplements have not necessarily been proven to reduce miscarriage, however it's probably a good idea to make sure your vitamin has selenium in it. Selenium has found to be most effective

---

[135] Abdulah R, Noerjasin H, Septiani L, Mutakin, Defi IR, Suradji EW, Puspitasari IM, Barliana MI, Yamazaki C, Nakazawa M, Koyama H.
Reduced serum selenium concentration in miscarriage incidence of Indonesian subjects.,Biol Trace Elem Res. 2013 Jul;154(1):1-6. doi: 10.1007/s12011-013-9701-0. Epub 2013 May 22.

when taken with magnesium, so check for both in your prenatal vitamin.

Zinc

Zinc deficiency can cause chromosomal changes in both men and women which could lead to miscarriage.

Omega-3

Aside from all of the benefits of omega-3's, there may be evidence that they can help prevent miscarriage. Pregnant women who take fish oil supplements may cut miscarriage risk due to inflammation of the placenta, and also improve the function of placenta.

As published in the Journal of Lipid Research, omega 3 fatty acids (fish Oil) affected the placenta and fetus of pregnant laboratory animals. After fish oil supplementation, the placenta had higher levels of compounds called resolvins. The study concluded that the omega-3 fatty acids present in fish oil can help limit inflammation in the placenta.[136]

Good news for Chocolate Lovers!

One study found that women who reported regular chocolate consumption of ≥1-3 servings/week had a 50% reduced risk of preeclampsia. Although this particular study did not separate out regular chocolate from dark chocolate, it is thought that theobromine, the bitter-tasting chemical in cocoa (in higher concentrations in dark

---

[136] Jones, M. L., Mark, P. J., Keelan, J. A., Barden, A., Mas, E., Mori, T. A., & Waddell, B. J. (2013). Maternal dietary omega-3 fatty acid intake increases resolvin and protectin levels in the rat placenta. Journal of lipid research, 54(8), 2247-2254.

chocolate), helps to regulate blood pressure by helping blood vessels to dilate.[137]

What does a miscarriage feel like? How do you know if you're having one?

After having six miscarriages, and going back and analyzing some of the signs and symptoms, I can share the following (at least from my experience):

- Spotting or bleeding during pregnancy was one of the first indicators. However, many normal pregnancies (including my successful pregnancy) have some implantation bleeding. So this may have to be evaluated along with other symptoms.
- Cramping (usually somewhat more severe than minor cramping) especially when accompanied by bleeding or even the passage of clots.
- A change in BBT (basal body temperature) - If you are monitoring your temperature, you may see a drop after a miscarriage.
- Sudden loss of pregnancy symptoms: this doesn't always happen, but one of my miscarriages did have a sudden loss of symptoms along with a gush of blood one morning.
- Pelvic pain sudden or progressive could be a sign of an ectopic pregnancy. I did have an ectopic pregnancy and from the very beginning I had a dull pelvic pain, but right before the surgery (after it was found on ultrasound), I had a sharp severe pain and it was in the process of rupturing when they removed it.

---

[137] Saftlas, A. F., Triche, E. W., Beydoun, H., & Bracken, M. B. (2010). Does Chocolate Intake During Pregnancy Reduce the Risks of Preeclampsia and Gestational Hypertension? Annals of Epidemiology, 20(8), 584–591. doi:10.1016/j.annepidem.2010.05.010

Chapter 13
"Do You Have Children??" How to Deal With All Those Tough Questions and Other Tough Situations

Every infertile couple has dealt with the inevitable "Do you have children?" or "When are you going to have kids?" questions. I know you feel like everyone out there is trying to jab a knife in your side, but for the fertile world it's a perfectly natural question to ask. No matter how many times it comes up, it seems like a total shock when the question comes hurling at you. Before I knew how to handle these inquiries, I would fumble around stuttering in embarrassment trying to come up with the right words to say. It would leave me feeling depressed for days. Part of managing your stress is being able to deal with these tough situations in a way that preserves your feelings.

Always anticipate the "having children" question will come up – especially when meeting someone new or when reconnecting with someone you haven't seen in a while. Remember, people are not trying to hurt your feelings. As a matter of fact, now that I have my daughter, I find myself asking others that question all the time. Even after everything I've been through, I don't automatically assume the person/couple might be having difficulty conceiving.

First let me tell you my response to the "having children" question:

"We got married later in life and by the time we really considered it, we felt we were on a different path."

Yes, I lied and a little white lie now and then is OK. The reason I gave this response is it seemed any other response would give people more information than I wanted to share. I really didn't want people to know I was trying to get pregnant because I was so sensitive about my age. I also found this response stopped this line of questioning dead in its tracks. If you do get pregnant and you see these people again, you can say, "what a pleasant surprise!" and you won't be lying!

Other responses I've heard include:

- We're trying
- Not yet
- Someday
- We can't
- Apparently not!
- We're very blessed with what we have
- Babies seem to come when they're good and ready
- When we decide (or when we get pregnant), you'll be the first to know!

Sharing Information

Everyone has to decide for themselves how public you want to be about your struggle with infertility. Some people tell nobody (like me), some people only tell close family and friends, and others tell anyone and everyone who will listen. Again, there is no right or wrong path to take when it comes to sharing information. You really have to do what helps you get through this ordeal. There are advantages and disadvantages either way. Consider the following before you decide who to share your information with:

If you share information about your struggle with infertility, others will know what questions *not* to ask, thereby avoiding uncomfortable situations. They will hopefully be more sensitive to your needs and they will be less likely to hurt your feelings with needless "kiddie" talk. This also gives you the opportunity to talk freely about your feelings and release some of your stress which can ultimately help you relax. The downside of telling others is they may purposefully avoid talking with you about certain subjects which can leave you feeling isolated and like somewhat of an outcast. To me, there would be nothing worse than finding out a mutual acquaintance is pregnant and then find out everyone was trying to keep it from me. I knew a woman who went through this very situation. She had a relative who became pregnant, but nobody told her and she wound up finding out at a family gathering. She broke down and cried in front of everyone because she just didn't have the opportunity to prepare. You also may feel like others are walking on eggshells around you which can be quite uncomfortable.

Another downside of sharing information is you may be excluded from certain social gatherings. For instance, you may not be invited to baby showers, kids' birthday parties, etc. Even though you may have *chosen* not attend to these events, it hurts when you are purposefully excluded. Most people who haven't gone through infertility can't possibly know how it feels and they don't know the right thing to do. If you do decide to share information with others, perhaps you need to tell them what you can and can't handle at the time.

Sharing information with co-workers can also be somewhat of a sticky wicket. Many women I've known who were trying to get pregnant did not want to tell anyone at work because they were afraid it would hurt their career if their employer knew they might get pregnant and go on maternity leave or quit. Additionally, sometimes people in a competitive work environment can use this information against you. I knew a manager who shared her struggle to get pregnant with her subordinates. A pregnant employee accused this manager of treating her worse than the other employees stating she was jealous. The moral of the story is: think before your share your personal and sensitive information. Once you share it, you can't take it back.

One more drawback of freely sharing information is people, although well meaning, might continually ask you if you've had any luck on the "pregnancy front". Or you may always feel like they're wondering why it's taking so long. I found it easier to fail in private rather than in public. Even though I knew deep down I would succeed, I didn't know how long it would take. For me, it helped to keep things to myself. Again, you must decide what works for you. It's a very individual thing.

Dealing With Fertile Friends & Relatives

Chances are you have friends and/or relatives who are having kids. I was somewhat fortunate that most of my immediate family is older than me and their kids were grown or practically grown by the time I started trying to get pregnant. However, it's hard to escape *someone* close getting pregnant before you. If it's not a family member, it might be a co-worker or other acquaintance. This situation is incredibly difficult for the infertile person/couple. Not only do you feel bad when someone announces they're pregnant, but you feel guilty for not being happy for them.

You're not a bad person for feeling this way. Almost all infertile people I've talked to have been through this emotional dilemma – it is perfectly normal and you should not add to your stress by feeling bad about it.

Here are some ways to deal with the tough situations that may come up from time to time:

Someone announces they're pregnant

Politely say "Congratulations, I know you'll be a great mom". Feel free to excuse yourself at the next available opportunity – even if it's a fake phone call or a trip to the bathroom.

Holiday gatherings include kids or a new baby

This might be the perfect opportunity to help in the kitchen. Again, if you can anticipate the difficult situation, you can prepare yourself which is half the battle. Be the first one to volunteer to clear the dishes and clean up. Also seating arrangements might be thought about ahead of time. Maybe sit next to older relatives who aren't into the "kiddie" talk. Be polite – acknowledge the babies/children, tell the parents how cute they are and how they've grown. You don't have to go on and on, but you'll probably feel better if you at least say *something* nice. If holidays are just too painful, perhaps going out of town might be the ticket. This is probably something you can't do every holiday, but at least it's an option during your really tough times.

You see pregnant people/babies everywhere

Running errands and shopping early in the morning or if possible, late in the evening or mealtimes usually minimizes your exposure to babies, families, etc.

Baby Showers

If you don't think you can handle a baby shower, send a gift and a card with your apologies that you had another engagement. Baby showers are tough because everyone talks about….what else? Having babies! Again, you need to take care of *you* right now. On the other hand, if you can get yourself in the right mindset, you might attend the shower knowing one day it will be your turn! You'll want everyone to be happy for you when you get pregnant and I found that all the people I was happy for (even if I had to force myself to be happy) gave me double the happiness when I finally succeeded.

You get infuriated by how other women take their pregnancy and/or children for granted

Oh yes, we've all been there – a co-worker, relative, friend, or just a casual acquaintance starts talking about how they're pregnant with their third child. "Gee, we already have two boys, we thought we'd try for a girl" *Just like that…huh?* I had an exercise instructor who was 7 months pregnant and said that as she's doing her jumping jacks with her pregnant belly bulging through her leotard. I almost got up and walked out. I wanted to tell her she was an ungrateful little #$%^*!!! In a situation like this, if you can, try to change the subject. I think I chimed in and asked her about the updated class schedule. You can always leave, but you don't want to be running from every situation. If you have enough coping mechanisms, you can get through anything. Remember, everyone is on their own path in life. Other women who seem to have it all probably have some other challenge they're dealing with (maybe they have problems with their kids!) I'm not saying you should take pleasure if they go through tough times, but it really does you no good to feel envious of someone else's life when you really can't know everything about their individual struggles.

People who stick their nose in your business

We've already talked about people who innocently ask if you have children but there are others who seem to persist. If you haven't been open about your struggle with infertility, some people might try to talk you into having children or they may go on and on about how you shouldn't wait too long. They also might go into how wonderful their children are and how they're the best thing in their life. I find the best way to deal with people like this is politely say "I guess when the time is right everything will fall into place". The other option is to go ahead and tell the person you are struggling with infertility. Beware, however, this might bring up other comments like "relax and it will happen", "have you seen a doctor?", or "have you considered adoption?"

While we're on the subject of people asking about adoption, let me say that although I've seen adoption work beautifully for many people, it was never an option for us. We couldn't deal with having a third party involved (i.e. the birth mother) and after struggling with fertility treatments for so long, we couldn't take another roller coaster ride. It was particularly infuriating when someone asked if we'd considered adoption. It's like they want to give you this neat, tidy, quick and easy solution to a very complicated issue. Additionally, for me, moving on to adoption meant I had failed. I had this deep knowing inside of me that if I persisted, I would succeed. I always had to resist the temptation to say, "Why don't *YOU* consider adoption?" – But of course I didn't. I had to remind myself that people really do just want to help.

Again, probably the best strategy in most of these situations is to change the subject as quickly as possible. As a matter of fact, if you know you're going to be seeing or speaking with a nosy friend or relative, you might think ahead of time about certain questions or subjects you can ask to redirect the conversation when things get on the wrong track. For example, if someone starts asking about whether or not you've decided to have children, you might say, "oh our lives are so busy right now ---- but, before I forget, I was going to ask you how your new job is going." Preparation is really the key to getting through tough situations. I found the worst part of any encounter of this nature was being unprepared.

If you have been open about trying to get pregnant, you may receive comments like, "Why would *anyone* want a baby at *your* age? It's selfish because you won't be around to raise them."

One of my speaking engagements was on a radio program discussing pregnancy over the age of 40. The radio host played "devil's advocate" by asking me some of these questions. Here's what I told him and his listeners:

"Statistically speaking, women who have their first child over the age of forty are four times more likely to live to be one hundred. It's thought that the surge of hormones in pregnancy have a rejuvenating effect on the body. Also, women who have children later in life have fewer pregnancies and that's less wear and tear on their body.

Women who have children at an older age are more motivated to take care of themselves which may also contribute to a longer life span."

Next time someone is rude enough to make a comment about being too old to have a baby, just politely inform them of the facts. Avoid the temptation to get angry or upset with others who unknowingly hurt your feelings or say the wrong thing. I know the feeling of being on the edge of saying something I would regret later. You have to remember *you* are hypersensitive right now and people in the fertile world just don't know how it feels just as you may not understand certain aspects of their life. If you say something rude or nasty to someone who makes a comment about getting pregnant, you will probably feel worse about yourself later which will add to your stress. It really is best to be polite, even if you have to leave the situation. I do recall a few times when it took everything I had in me to keep my mouth in check—but I was always happy I did.

Another infertile friend gets pregnant before you

The reason I bring this up is because I previously talked about joining a support group. Most women in the support group will eventually succeed (as will you!) You'll feel a little pang of "why not me?" when others announce they are pregnant before you. It's much easier to handle because you know they've been through the same struggle you have and you know they don't take their pregnancy for granted. The way I chose to handle this is to see others' success as a glimmer of hope. I honestly think that's one reason I did finally succeed – I saw other women succeed and it proved to me it *can* be done. Remember, you need to treat them the way you want them to treat you when you succeed. Be happy for them! Their success is your success because it will ultimately show you there is light at the end of the struggle. Congratulate them and remember one day you may be raising your kids together. I still stay in touch with many of the women I met in the support group. We had play dates when the kids were younger, we went to birthday parties and we are all friends on social media sites. It's a reminder of how far we've all come. I can't tell you how many times I've heard women who struggled with infertility (and eventually got pregnant) say, "If *I* can get pregnant, *anybody* can!" It just goes to show you everyone going through infertility feels this may be an impossible dream from time to time. So many of us succeeded and *you* are no different. You deserve everything life has to offer just as much as anyone else.

Part II

My Infertility and Miscarriage Story

Chapter 14
How Did It Come To This? How My Past Experiences and Choices Led to Infertility

Getting married and having children was never a goal of mine, as a matter of fact, it was something I really wanted to avoid. I grew up in a family where I was the youngest of three girls and had parents who were quite mismatched. My parents were primarily motivated by making money and I was put in daycare so my mother could work full time. To this day, daycare was probably the worst experience of my whole life at a time when I was the least able to handle it. My mother seemed to be totally overwhelmed with life in general and I was at the bottom of her priority list. My job in the family was to stay out of the way. I watched my mother shower her attention (what little there was of it) on my older sisters who always had the luxury of some crisis going on. As a result I became a very disagreeable child (only at home – outside the house, I was an angel). It's no wonder I viewed marriage and children as the plague to be avoided at all costs. Even though I had many friends and was a good student, I had very low self-esteem. I never had the benefit of a mother and father who took an interest in me or had the time to devote to a third child. I had the distinct impression I wasn't worth the time or attention my sisters were entitled to.

I didn't get married until I was 36 years old. In my 20's, unlike most of my peers, I had no desire to settle down. The thought of marriage and kids felt like a noose around my neck. I dated, but I seemed to attract men that were about as uncommitted as I was. I filled my time with a high stress management position in a large healthcare organization while simultaneously working on my MBA. I started working in middle management when I was 22 years old, right out of college. My goal was to be a high powered corporate executive making a lot of money and living the high life. I wanted the best of everything and had a desire to impress those around me.

I was 28 years old when I had a gynecological exam and was told I had some uterine fibroids. My doctor explained what a fibroid was and how it could eventually affect fertility. Hey, no big deal – who wanted kids anyway? I ignored the fibroids and I didn't go in for routine annual exams, mainly because I was young and usually too busy to fit it in. When I was 31, however, I started to have some slight pelvic pain which would shoot down my right leg. I decided to have it checked out. The fibroids I ignored had grown significantly and were continuing to grow quite fast. I underwent major abdominal surgery to have my fibroids removed at the age of 31. The recovery was about six weeks and I went on with my usual high stress life. A few years later, my gynecologist found a new fibroid, but it was small and we decided to just keep an eye on it. I absolutely did not want to go through surgery again.

When I was 34, I met the man I eventually married. I didn't think it was possible for me to commit to anyone, but I guess when you find the right person, it's quite easy. We married two years later and initially we decided not to have children. However, when I started becoming disillusioned with the corporate world, the idea of having a child and staying home to raise him/her started to sound quite appealing. The corporate world was becoming so cut-throat, it was hard to get up and go to work each day. I saw people who had worked their entire life for the company get laid off on a whim. I really wanted a more simple life. The older I got, the more I realized that having children could be a very loving and rewarding experience. Family life didn't have to be a bad thing. I began to notice babies everywhere – I longed for my own. My husband and I both agreed we would start trying to have a child about seven months after we were married. I was 37.

Somewhere in the back of my mind, maybe because of my past surgery, I thought I might have trouble conceiving. I even recall a time when I was engaged and someone asked if we were going to have children. I jokingly said, "Oh, I'm probably infertile - Ha Ha!" I had no idea what I was in for. The optimistic side of me thought once we started trying, we would be pregnant right away. I never thought my age was a factor (I'm still not convinced it was) – I considered myself young and healthy. It's almost funny now to think about, but the first time we had intercourse without the use of birth control, we were planning my maternity leave and how we would fit a baby into our lives. Of course, those were the days before I had "period calendars" where my menstrual cycle was mapped out for the two magic ovulation days and intercourse was mandatory.

As each month went by, I began to get a sinking feeling in my gut that perhaps my earlier comments about being infertile weren't so far off the mark. After about seven months of trying, and after my 38th birthday, I made an appointment with my primary care doctor with the intention of getting a referral to an RE (reproductive endocrinologist). I knew about reproductive endocrinology because my original fibroid surgery was done by an RE. Maybe subconsciously I went to him because I wanted to preserve my fertility. It took a few months to get an appointment with a RE and that coincided with the one year "trying to get pregnant" mark, which is most doctors' definition of infertility.

We told absolutely no one we were trying to get pregnant or that we were seeing a fertility doctor. I didn't want any of my single, childless friends to know because I thought they'd think I was going to abandon them. I didn't tell my family and my husband didn't tell his

Chapter 15
My Experience with Assisted Reproductive Technologies

We met with a reproductive endocrinologist shortly after my 38th birthday and we went through my husband's history and my history. The RE zeroed in on my past surgery and a new problem: I had started spotting between periods. We immediately did all lab work and it showed my FSH was about 7 which is in the normal range. They tested my progesterone and it was shown to be a bit low in the second half of my cycle. We also did a post-coital test where you have intercourse in the evening and the next morning they check the condition of the sperm. This test tells you whether or not you have "hostile" cervical mucus (i.e. your cervical mucus is not "sperm friendly") and the results were somewhat abnormal as well. Additionally, my RE wanted to do an exploratory laparoscopy and a hysteroscopy to see if he could find out why I was spotting between periods. That surgery was quite minor, but productive. He found a small fibroid (probably the one I ignored years ago) and polyp which were removed. He found a few areas of endometriosis which he removed as well. He checked my fallopian tubes with an HSG (a procedure where they inject dye in through your fallopian tubes) and found them to be open.

After the laparoscopy and hysteroscopy, I had to wait three months to heal, and then he recommended doing artificial insemination (with my husband's sperm) to bypass the hostile cervical environment. I also received hCG (the pregnancy hormone) shots after the insemination which stimulates the ovaries to produce progesterone to build up and maintain the uterine lining. My husband's sperm count was excellent (in the billions) so at the very least we didn't have to worry about that. We tried 3 months of inseminations with no results and then my doctor decided to try Clomid. We tried inseminations with Clomid for the next 4 months with no results. I certainly was ovulating because we'd check how many follicles were visible on ultrasound and I would sometimes have up to five. No one knew why I wasn't conceiving. As a matter of fact, my diagnosis was technically "unexplained infertility."

We met with our doctor again, and decided it was time to take the next step and try IVF. I was 39 (almost 40) at this point. The thought of going through IVF was scary! After all, I was graduating from high school when the first "test tube" baby was born (and they actually *did* call it a test tube baby back then!) I thought that was mad science at the time and here I was about to go through it! Even though I knew there were going to be more shots and procedures, I was excited to move on to the next step. Something was going to work eventually, right? At this point I decided it was time to quit my high stress job. I couldn't imagine going through the rigors of IVF *and* working the long hours that were expected of me at work.

Our first IVF cycle was pretty much what I thought it would be. We learned about all the drugs I had to take (my husband had to learn how to give me injections) and a couple of weeks later we went in for the egg retrieval. I was very nervous but everything went wonderfully. I had 18 good eggs retrieved – apparently, that's quite a successful cycle at my age. The embryologist mixed the eggs with my husband's sperm and we waited 3 days before going back for the embryo transfer. We had 5 good embryos. All 5 were transferred and the waiting game began. I had my blood drawn ten days after the transfer and again 2 days later so they could check if I had a positive hCG level (the second blood draw is especially important – if you are pregnant, the second blood draw shows whether or not the numbers are doubling like they should). Normally they don't call you until after the results of the second blood draw are in. But surprisingly, I received a phone call the afternoon of the first blood draw. The nurse started the conversation with "Congratulations". I was stunned. I thought it was too soon to know if I was really pregnant since the second blood draw had not been done. The nurse told me my hCG numbers were quite high and there could even be more than one embryo implanted. I was in disbelief…I didn't know if I should be too excited or not. There was still a long way to go. The second blood test confirmed the first and showed the numbers were indeed doubling. There was nothing to do but wait at this point since the first ultrasound isn't done until approximately 6 weeks gestation.

I was very nauseated throughout the entire 6 weeks before my ultrasound. I was also very tired and very nervous. I had what they called "hyperstimulation" of my ovaries, which can happen when you take fertility drugs. This created a little pelvic pain and pressure, however hyperstimulation can sometimes lead to serious complications. The day of our first ultrasound, I was excited but nervous. I had some spotting on and off, but the office assured me spotting was quite common especially with IVF patients. When it was time for the ultrasound, my heart was beating so fast and hard, I was sure everyone could hear and see it. The ultrasound technician inserted the vaginal probe and immediately blurts out "Oh, you have an ectopic!" She then said, "I see another one in your uterus, but I don't see a heartbeat." I was a little shell shocked and kind of stared at her in disbelief. "What do we do now?" I said. She got a very nervous look on her face and ran for the door saying "I need to get the doctor". I immediately started crying because I knew enough to know I did not have a viable pregnancy and the ectopic had to be removed surgically. The doctor made the quickest entrance I'd ever seen. The ultrasound tech must have yanked him away from another patient. He came in and did an ultrasound himself and confirmed the worst. He said I had a tubal pregnancy and an intrauterine pregnancy with no heartbeat. He said he'd been practicing for 25 years and had never seen a patient with both an ectopic and a failed intrauterine pregnancy. *Ok, now I'm a freak.*

I went into surgery that evening. Ectopic pregnancies are considered quite urgent as they can actually be life threatening if they rupture. The worst part was we had to tell both our families (I guess we didn't have to, but if something had gone wrong in surgery, it would have been a very difficult situation). We never told our families we had gone through IVF, and we never told them I had lost twins, but now they knew we were trying to get pregnant which I would have preferred to keep private. I had a surgical left salpingectomy (removal of my left tube) and a D & C to remove the uterine pregnancy. Fortunately, the tubal pregnancy was removed laparoscopically which reduced my recovery time.

I had my post-surgical visit and I told my doctor I wanted to try again. I had to wait 3 months for everything to heal. That three months seemed like an eternity. Not only was I mourning the loss of two babies, but I felt like I was going through a serious post-partum depression. I cried and cried until I could cry no more. After my hormones leveled out and I got my feet back on the ground, we were ready for the second try. The second IVF cycle was pretty much like the first. We already knew about the medications, the shots, and the general IVF protocol. It was now December and I was ready to get moving. It was a couple of weeks before Christmas when we started up with the shots. I had my egg retrieval and embryo transfer without incident. This time, we let the embryos grow to the blastocyst stage. This was somewhat of a new technique (at the time). If embryos grow to the blastocyst stage, you can see which ones survive the longest allowing you to implant only the best (reducing the chance of multiple births). We had three good embryos and all were implanted.

Then came the agonizing wait. I had my blood drawn ten days after the procedure and again two days later. After my second blood draw, I was sitting by the phone all day waiting, waiting, and waiting. I was surprised I didn't get a call that afternoon especially since I was called so quickly after my first IVF. Finally at about 4:30pm, I still had no word and I was afraid the office had forgotten to call me. I decided to call and they said they would give my message to the nurse. I was so stressed out and so angry at this point! Don't these people realize what their patients are going through??? I started to get a real sinking feeling in my gut. If they had good news, they probably would have called me right away. About 15 minutes later the phone rang. It was the fertility clinic nurse. She never said whether or not I was pregnant, she just rambled about what the numbers were. Apparently, I did have a positive hCG test, but she said it didn't double. So now what?? She said to come in 48 hours later for another blood draw. I promptly ended the conversation and called my husband sobbing hysterically. I knew we had failed again. *Merry Christmas....*

My next blood draw showed the numbers were going up, but they still hadn't doubled. After more lab work, the nurse told me point blank this was not a viable pregnancy and it was behaving like an ectopic. *Oh God, here we go again. What a cruel universe we live in.* I knew about a drug called methotrexate which could help expel the pregnancy without surgery (after all, I only had one tube left) and I told her I wanted it as soon as possible. If I wasn't pregnant, I wanted everything out of me now! She agreed and got orders for this medication. I went into the office, received a shot and I started bleeding (like a regular period) a week later. We checked my hCG's until they returned to zero.

My husband and I decided at this point we were through! Damn the doctors, damn the nurses, damn the drugs, and damn all the women with their big happy families. On top of all of that I had to endure the holidays with everyone "making merry". That gives you a sense of my frame of mind at this point. I wrote a letter to the fertility clinic explaining our decision to end fertility treatments, and I received a letter back telling me I was in the "resolution" phase of my infertility. *What the hell did that mean?* It didn't matter, I was never going to see any of them again. The nurse did tell me to use birth control for at least 3 months after taking methotrexate because you should not get pregnant while it's in your system due to the chance of birth defects (yeah, I thought, like *that's* really going to happen).

I was finished having my life controlled by a bunch of insensitive nurses and office staff and I could start thinking about moving on. My husband and I started to realize that despite a few close calls, we may never be parents. We just had waited too long and my previous high stress lifestyle had taken a toll on my reproductive system.

Even after all that, I still had this little voice in the back of my head saying *"You can still get pregnant, you're just on the wrong path"*. I got to thinking – I still have one tube, what if I could get pregnant naturally? This would be on *my* terms, not some high tech assembly line fertility clinic protocol. After all, both of my grandmothers had babies over 40 – and I was related to them (I don't think my parents had sex after I was born, so I guess my mother didn't count). I must have a good egg in there somewhere! I had this gut level feeling I *could* get pregnant and I could do it the old fashioned way. My body functioned well in every other way, and I still had all (or most) of my reproductive parts with the exception of my left tube.

As if to spur me on, I kept hearing about women in their 40's who got pregnant without fertility treatments. It seemed like all of a sudden, no matter where I went or who I talked to, I would hear about another woman giving birth in her forties. A tenant in our rental property told me she had given birth to her son when she was 44. A local radio personality talked about how his mother gave birth to him when she was 48 (before the days of fertility treatments.) I overheard some people talking in the ski lift line about how their mother had a baby at 43. I met another woman who had a baby naturally at 44 (after 4 miscarriages). I went to my niece's graduation party and I met a mother of triplets who conceived naturally and gave birth to them at the age of 45! I knew it could be done, I had living proof! I knew I could become pregnant and have a baby – *I just knew it.*

I started looking for a part-time job (mostly to pass the time until I became pregnant), and began teaching a couple of classes at the local community college. I guess that master's degree was good for something! I really didn't want to go back working in the corporate world – that was an unhealthy and stressful lifestyle. The one good thing about being older was we were financially secure and I didn't have to work. Teaching was something I enjoyed and it was good to have something to do other than thinking about getting pregnant.

I began my new journey, but this time it would be on *my* terms.

Chapter 16
My Experience with Recurrent Miscarriage

I had a harder journey than most when it comes to miscarriage - I had six of them. The first three were the end result of my fertility treatments. My first IVF resulted in the loss of twins (one was ectopic, one died in my uterus – both were quite early in the pregnancy). My third pregnancy loss was after the second IVF where my hCG numbers were not doubling and they strongly suspected another ectopic. Fortunately, I was able to take methotrexate to expel the second ectopic pregnancy rather than going through another surgery. This also preserved the only tube I had left which was my only chance at succeeding naturally.

About 9 months after completing our fertility treatments (and 9 months after my second ectopic) I started having some irregular bleeding. I remember thinking it was an odd time to have a period. My legs felt very tired and I felt very crampy. I thought I was having a period, but it was very light (my periods have been very light for over 10 years, but this was exceptionally light). I remember my breasts were also sore which was somewhat unusual. It dawned on me I might be pregnant. I went and got a home pregnancy test and sure enough, it came out positive. I was absolutely shocked! I called the doctor's office and told them I had a positive test but I was bleeding and I had a history of 2 ectopics. Since it was a Friday afternoon, they told me to go to the ER since I was at higher risk of having an ectopic which could be life threatening.

My visit to the ER was interesting – I'm sure ER doctors are generally good at what they do, but they certainly are not good at reading vaginal ultrasounds! I wound up having a catheter inserted (to inflate my bladder) and I had to go to Radiology for an abdominal and vaginal ultrasound. Basically, they said it was not a viable pregnancy and what they saw was a collapsed gestational sac. Believe it or not, I was not even upset. I was actually happy I got pregnant on my own! Even though I lost this pregnancy, it showed me I was capable of getting pregnant, even with one tube! The ER staff tried to console me and I kept telling them, "Hey, it's ok…this is actually good news for me." Since I'm Rh negative, they gave me a Rhogam shot, and I was on my way. I started bleeding and passed some tissue about 5 weeks later. We continued to check my hCG's until they returned to "0".

Now… back to the drawing board.

I continued on with my healthy diet and I was now more motivated than ever. Even though this miscarriage was a tough break, I now *knew* without a doubt I could get pregnant on my own without fertility treatments. Then, about 8 months later, I noticed my period had not come by day 27 (usually I would have it by now), so I did a pregnancy test. It was negative. I started having some brown spotting, but I still did not have my period by day 28, so I did another test, but this time it was positive. I was so happy! I really thought this pregnancy would make it. I called my OB right away and since I had a bad pregnancy history, we started monitoring my hCG's (mainly to rule out an ectopic). My hCG's looked good, they were more than doubling every 48 hours. I actually started to get morning sickness. We decided to do an ultrasound when my hCG's were over 2000 since this is the time you're able to visualize something. We did determine it was an intrauterine pregnancy (not ectopic), but all we could see was a yolk sac and a fetal pole. They told me to come back in a week since it was so early in the pregnancy that a week would make a big difference. I went back a week later. This time we did another ultrasound and we saw a heartbeat. The ultrasound was done by a PA, so she went to get the doctor just to double check if everything was where it should be. The doctor came right in the room, but the first thing he said was "the heartbeat is slow". I don't know how fast it was beating – but it looked fine to me. He told me I was at risk of miscarriage since the heartbeat was so slow. He said it wasn't inevitable, but there certainly was a threat.

I was very upset after I left the office. I had told my whole family I was pregnant, and now I was at risk of losing my baby. Later that week, I had a small gush of blood and I felt less nauseated. *Not a good sign.* I knew immediately there was a problem, and coupled with the fact that there was a slow heartbeat a week earlier, I prepared myself for the worst.

I went back to the office a week later, and another ultrasound confirmed my worst fears. The heart had stopped beating. Why was this happening to me??? I finally get pregnant (twice!) on my own and now I have to deal with repeatedly miscarrying my pregnancies. I had a good cry and I asked my husband to let my family know about the situation. My doctor decided to see if the pregnancy would expel on its own, but after 3 weeks of constant nausea and hCG's that weren't decreasing significantly, we decided to do a D & C. I asked to have the fetal tissue genetically tested to see if there was a chromosomal abnormality. After the D & C, I immediately felt better (as far as being nauseated). The results of the genetic testing came back and the fetus was a chromosomally *normal* boy. The doctor said it was probably a poor attachment that caused the problems.

I went on my way but believe it or not, I was just as motivated to try again. If I could get pregnant twice on my own and have a chromosomally normal baby, I just knew I could succeed. I picked myself up by my bootstraps and decided to keep on trying.

After this last miscarriage, I decided to have another hysteroscopy, just to see if I had a new fibroid or something that might be interfering with the implantation. My hysteroscopy was done by a reproductive endocrinologist and everything looked clean as a whistle in my uterus. *Wouldn't you know it?!* In some ways this was good news, but in other ways it was quite frustrating because nobody could tell me why I couldn't carry a baby to term! I guess infertility was not my problem now, miscarriage was. But hey, the bottom line was I didn't have a baby – for whatever reason. I decided I would just keep plugging along. I knew I could get pregnant with a normal child and it was just a matter of getting that pregnancy to attach properly. I decided to visualize and meditate on a secure attachment. I continued with my healthy diet and the other treatments in my pregnancy protocol.

About 5 months later I started having some strange brown spotting – similar to the spotting I had with previous pregnancies. I kind of knew the routine by now, so I did a pregnancy test around day 28. Sure enough, it was positive. I was a bit hesitant to get excited this time so I kept my emotions under control. I called the doctor's office – they ordered my hCG's. The first one came out fine, but again, it's whether or not they're doubling that counts. I had the second hCG drawn a few days later. They called me back and said it didn't quite double so they wanted to wait two more days and evaluate the numbers. I started to get a sinking feeling. Could this possibly be happening again??? NO! I started to prepare myself for the worst. I had another hCG drawn and they called me back and sheepishly told me the hCG's didn't do anything. The numbers stayed flat. This was not a viable pregnancy. They told me I would probably start bleeding soon and I should get another Rhogam shot when I started bleeding. I thanked them, I cried for 15 minutes and I told myself I needed to look at this as just a late period. I started bleeding about 2 weeks later and I had a very strong Manhattan (I know I said not to drink alcohol, but hey, there are benefits to not being pregnant and at this point I needed a strong one!)

OK, now what? Did I have it in me to keep trying? I knew I couldn't let go. It seemed the older I got, the more I got pregnant on my own. *One has got to stick eventually!*

Chapter 17
Success at Last!

It's when lower your resistance you finally succeed!

It had been about a year since my last miscarriage and I had not conceived again. I religiously attended my support group for which I was the leader. The constant disappointment of not getting pregnant every month was starting to wear on me and since my 44th birthday was approaching, I was feeling the need to move on with my life. I resigned as the support group leader and decided to move on to "childfree". It wasn't an easy decision, and after much private screaming and crying, I accepted defeat. I made peace with the fact that I just wasn't going to have children. I tried to focus on all of the positive aspects of my life and all of the things I would be able to do living a childfree lifestyle. For the first time in six years, I felt a heavy weight was lifted off my shoulders and my mind felt open to do something else besides trying to get pregnant. I was tired but relieved to have made such a big decision. Now....time to move forward with the rest of my life.

A couple of weeks after my last support group meeting, for once, I wasn't paying attention to when my period was supposed to start but it seemed like it was about due. It was about day 26 of my September menstrual cycle and this was usually was when I would start to have a little spotting like my period was on the way (my cycles at this time were about 26-28 days). On a whim, I searched through my bathroom cabinet for a pregnancy test. Like most women who have experienced infertility, I always had at least one "just in case". The one that I had was supposedly able to detect as little as 20 mIU/ml hCG in your system (some brands require 100 mIU/ml hCG). When I did the test, there was a *very* faint line indicating I was pregnant. I actually looked at it through a magnifying glass and sure enough, it was positive. I thought maybe the test was invalid since I'd had it so long in my cabinet (even though it was still within its expiration date.) I didn't say anything to my husband and I went to the store and bought another pregnancy test just to confirm (especially since the line was so faint). I waited two more days before I did the second test, and sure enough, it came out positive too…part of me thought…*yeah, right…playing tricks on me again?* It seemed so ironic that I was truly at peace with my decision to go childfree and here I was, back on the rollercoaster.

I don't know what my feelings were at this point. In many ways I was so excited I actually had gotten pregnant again, but in other ways I was just waiting for the miscarriage to happen. I finally told my husband after the second pregnancy test and his response was "Well, let's wait 9 months and see what happens". I actually got quite angry with him. Here I had spent the last 6 years of my life trying to get pregnant, and this is the response I get? He later apologized and told me what I was already feeling myself. How can you continually get excited about something that inevitably winds up being a major disappointment? I had to admit, I was really holding myself back from getting excited about this pregnancy too. It was so early and we had so far to go. It seemed the road to having a baby was filled with landmines and we had only dodged the first one. There were so many more out there waiting to trip us up.

I made the decision not to call my doctor. I absolutely didn't want the stress of going in every 48 hours for blood work

and then waiting for the bomb to drop. It was a
empowering to have this be *my* pregnancy
secret that nobody could take away from me. I fig
worst thing that could happen was I would have another ectopic and the chances were quite low. If I felt any sharp pains, I would go to the ER (since ectopics can be life threatening). I was going to treat this pregnancy like a normal person would. I would just let it happen and if I started bleeding, I would know I was having another miscarriage.

I immediately started to feel a little queasy, hmmm, that's a good sign. I had never felt sick this quickly before. I had read morning sickness is a good sign since it can mean your hormones are strong. I had also heard older women experience less morning sickness since they typically have lower hormone levels, and here I was, almost 44, already feeling sick! I started to feel some breast tenderness – another good sign. A few days after I took the pregnancy test, I had some dark brown spotting, *oh no…not a good sign.* I figured I would just let nature take its course. If I was going to lose this pregnancy, then so be it. I had all my defense mechanisms in place and I was not going to be the victim of any more cruelty.

I tried to take it easy. If I was going to miscarry, there was probably nothing I could do to stop it. I had read that bed rest had not shown to be beneficial in stopping miscarriage, but I was too scared to do any sort of physical exertion. About 10 days after my positive pregnancy test, I started to get *really* sick. I began vomiting and the nausea was so intense, it almost felt like I had the flu and a fever. As a matter of fact, I kept taking my temperature because I was sure this achy feeling must mean something else is going on. My temperature was normal. I just rested and kept eating at regular intervals to reduce the nausea. Speaking of eating, it seems I couldn't get enough food. I was always hungry. I had to have my husband keep going to the store to get more for me to eat. Also, I found eggnog had just come in season, and at 3:00am, it was a quick fix to reduce the nausea.

About 7 weeks had gone by and I still had some spotting (still that dark brown stuff). We kept the pregnancy secret and told absolutely no one. I secretly thought this would jinx my luck. I figured I did not have an ectopic because it probably would have ruptured by now and I knew my symptoms would not be as severe if this pregnancy was outside my uterus. I was literally bedridden with sickness at this point. I finally broke down and decided to call my doctor's office to let them know I was pregnant and to see if I could get an ultrasound. As much as I didn't want any bad news, I was really dying to know what was going on in there and I was far enough along that everything should be visible on an ultrasound. I called on Monday and they told me to come in the next morning at 8:00am (I always knew they would see me right away since I had a history of 2 ectopics).

The next morning came rolling around and my husband took time off work to go with me. I can't put into words how absolutely petrified I was to go to this appointment. I just knew I was going to be disappointed, crying, angry and so let down. *Why hadn't I just gone on birth control so I didn't have to go through this again?* My husband kept reassuring me he would be there and we'd get through this no matter what happened. Besides, if it wasn't a viable pregnancy, I would have to deal with it sooner or later and it might as well be sooner.

I walked in the doctor's office and I was literally shaking. My nervousness worsened my nausea and thankfully I brought some crackers with me. I played out the different scenarios in my mind. What would I say when they tell me it's not a viable pregnancy? Am I going to scream and cry or just sit there emotionless? Is there *any* possibility they would give me *good* news? I couldn't imagine it. At that moment, I felt like I was on trial waiting for the jury's verdict to be read.

The nurse finally called my name and I wasn't sure I could get up and walk to the exam room. Between my nausea and shaking, I actually felt like I was going to collapse. My heart was beating so hard and fast I was afraid I would miscarry just from the stress. I got on the ultrasound table and resisted the urge to get up and run out. I was so glad they didn't take my blood pressure because I was probably at the stroke level. The doctor came in and I told him I was very nervous about what we would find. He just said "well let's take a look". He inserted the vaginal probe ultrasound and I examined his face for any inkling of information. All of a sudden he blurts out "There's your pregnancy – and there's the heartbeat! It looks great! Wow, this is your time!" I sat there absolutely stunned. Surely there was some mistake. For a moment, in my fear and paranoia, I thought this was some secret plot or conspiracy against me. I could not believe my ears. Here was a doctor, usually quite composed, absolutely bouncing off the walls! It was the first time in six years, after six miscarriages that I ever heard *anything* positive from a gynecologist or OB doctor and this was over the top! I almost went into my *"I'm OK, this isn't the first time"* rhetoric (as if I needed to make *him* feel better for giving me the dreaded news.) Instead, I was hearing these magical words and I had not rehearsed what to say. I can't remember what I muttered, but whatever it was, it didn't do the situation justice. I was fighting back the tears, but these were tears of relief and dare I say joy?

This particular doctor was actually the RE who had previously done my hysteroscopy, so now that I was pregnant, he referred me to a regular OB. Imagine that, a *regular* OB! Before leaving the exam room, we all said our good byes and many "congratulations" later, we made our way back through the waiting area. There were many couples sitting there as we zig zagged through the maze of chairs. One of the difficult things about being in a RE's office is everyone knows why you're there. I could see some of them sneaking a glimpse of us out of the corner of my eye. They had no idea what kind of war stories we could tell. I could see the frustration on their faces and I felt a slight pang of guilt knowing I had this awesome secret hidden deep inside of me. I knew I had to stifle my excitement and put on my poker face as we went by, but part of me wanted to climb on the counter and scream "I'M PREGNANT!"

It was a quiet ride home, both of us replaying the wonderful sequence of events in our minds. I still didn't have the words to express what I felt. For the first time in a long time, perhaps ever, I felt totally at peace. I *knew* I had succeeded. This pregnancy was going to make it. When we got home, I ran in and threw up. But I can't tell you how happy I was, vomit and all.

I was about 9 1/2 weeks when I had my next doctor's visit. This is what "normal" people would call their first OB appointment. I was still having some spotting, and I was still very sick. My doctor decided to do another ultrasound since I had such a bad pregnancy history behind me. We all wanted to see what was going on even though I was still very scared to hear bad news. This ultrasound looked great! We could see a very strong heartbeat, we could see buds for the arms and legs, and we actually saw the baby move. I swear I could feel something moving inside of me, but they told me I wouldn't be able to feel the baby move until later. We saw a little blood between the gestational sac and my uterus. I was told this is nothing to worry about and it was probably the cause of my spotting. It was old blood from the implantation and since it was trapped between the uterus and the gestational sac, it was just coming out very slowly. We could still see a small portion of the yolk sac. I was told this is why I was feeling such nausea. As the fetus grows and the yolk sac disappears, the nausea usually goes away (about 12 weeks).

About two more weeks went by and my nausea started to subside. Oh, what a relief! Believe me, I wasn't complaining, but having been bedridden for all this time was very difficult. At our next appointment, we talked to the doctor about doing an amniocentesis. We made an appointment to have it done at about 15 weeks. *This was our next big hurdle.* Having an amnio is a double edged sword. On one hand, it can put your mind at ease because you worry about whether or not everything is ok --- especially at my age where the rate of chromosomal abnormalities is higher than for younger women. On the other hand, you worry about getting the results – *what if...* I couldn't even go there.

The day of our amniocentesis came around and I was still pregnant! Wow, 15 weeks! Definitely a new record for me. We still had not told anyone I was pregnant. We wanted the results of the amnio first. We went to a perinatologist who had done thousands of amnios – we only wanted the best. We saw a genetic counselor first who asked us a few questions about our backgrounds and a few questions about my pregnancy history. She said I did have a somewhat higher risk of chromosomal problems not only because of my age, but also because many miscarriages are due to chromosomal problems and it's nature's way of dealing with it. The counselor was very professional and explained the procedure and what the results would look like. The bad thing was we had to wait 14 days for the results. Apparently they have to grow the chromosomes, etc.

I went into the room where the amniocentesis was going to be performed. There is a special ultrasound machine which helps the physician guide the needle. I was extremely nervous because there is a small risk of miscarriage with an amnio and things had just gone so well up until this point. I didn't want to blow it now. Thankfully, the doctor had a wonderful bedside manner. He actually was making me laugh which I had to stop because I didn't want my belly shaking. When he was ready to insert the needle, I covered my eyes and ears and hummed. I know that sounds a little crazy, but it really helped to distract me from what was going on. The amnio did not hurt at all. I've had blood draws that were more painful than that! It was over in less than a minute. The doctor took two tubes of amniotic fluid out and then put a little band aid on my belly. I was told not to do anything strenuous for the rest of the day and that was it! I didn't have any cramping or anything. It was so easy! I really had worried for nothing. Prior to the amnio, I had a very detailed ultrasound where they measure the baby and they look to see if all of the organs are developing normally. Everything looked great! The doctor also told me sometimes there are "markers" for Down Syndrome that can be visualized on an ultrasound and he said he didn't see anything abnormal. He gave us some very nice ultrasound pictures and we were on our way. Now it was a waiting game for the results. They assured me they would call and keep calling until they were able to reach me as soon as the results were in.

Since I had been through so much, we decided my husband would take the call when it came. About 10 days later, the phone rang and I picked it up without looking at the caller ID. When the genetic counselor identified herself, I wanted to hang up and run away. I could feel all the old familiar feelings of dread welling up in me. The results were in. The first thing I said was *"Oh God...Do I want to talk to you?"* She said "You most certainly do! Everything is normal!" I was still in my dread mode and my heart was pounding. I could not believe I was getting more good news! She asked if I wanted to know the sex of the baby since we were unable to tell during the ultrasound. I emphatically said *"yes!"* but to be honest, I hadn't processed that I was actually going to have a baby. She said "It's a girl!" Wow! A girl! I was beyond happy but still in disbelief. Don't get me wrong, I would have been equally happy with a boy, but I grew up as a 'girly girl'. This was just a bonus. This truly was one of the best days of my life up until that point. It was December and Christmas was right around the corner. We were able to tell our families now. I was starting to show and I couldn't keep it a secret any longer. This was actually the first holiday season in over 6 years that I wasn't struggling with getting pregnant.

I immediately called my husband at work to tell him the news. He was surprised the results were in so quickly. We both figured they tell you it's going to take two weeks so you're pleasantly surprised when the results come back quicker. My husband was so pleased. Like me, he was very unaccustomed to getting good news. You almost get to the point where you've got so many defense mechanisms in place from dealing with the constant disappointment, you don't know if you dare get excited. By the end of the call I could hear the excitement and joy in his voice. This really was going to happen!

That evening, I called my mom. I said, "Guess what?" She said "What?" I said "Guess". She said "You're pregnant?" I said "Yep, I'm over 4 months!" She was soooo happy. Actually my family only knew about three of the miscarriages, so they didn't know how seemingly hopeless my situation was. They didn't even know we were trying to

:gnant anymore – and officially, we weren't. My
ıd called all of his relatives and I sent everyone e-mails
ultrasound which I scanned in my computer. This was
going to be a great holiday season. I'm normally not a
"holiday" person, but I was so happy to be finally on my way
to parenthood.

I decided to get back in touch with the women's infertility
support group to share my news. A number of people had
already gotten pregnant by then. They were truly happy for
me and I let them know I didn't break the group leader
winning streak. Later, I found out the group leader at the
time also got pregnant naturally at the age of 43 (she had her
baby at 44). She had been going through fertility treatments,
but decided to take a break. She got pregnant during her
break! See? This really *can* happen, not just to me.

The rest of my pregnancy was quite uneventful. I did have
another episode of spotting at about 26 weeks, but it turned
out to be nothing (probably a yeast infection which is quite
common in pregnancy). I had read once women with
infertility and miscarriage are also at risk for premature
delivery. I asked my doctor about this and she said she did
not have any reason to think I would deliver prematurely. I
guess I kept thinking something was going to go wrong.
That's just one of those realities when you've dealt with so
many failures.

I had always envisioned myself as someone who would be
very physically active during pregnancy. The truth of the
matter is I spent a good part of my pregnancy lying on my
left side with my feet elevated. I had read many miscarriages
(or premature deliveries) could be prevented by keeping
your feet elevated which takes pressure off your cervix.
Lying on your left side supposedly is the best position to
deliver blood flow and oxygen to your baby. I had no

medical reason to be worried, but I figured I wanted to take every precaution I could.

All throughout my pregnancy, I continued with my healthy diet and drank 64-80 oz of water per day. The only thing I did differently is I ate more protein. I almost had to do this because I was so hungry all the time. I must say, however, during the first trimester when my morning sickness was at its peak, I ate whatever made the nausea subside. That usually included many creamy or starchy foods like ice cream, egg nog, mashed potatoes and gravy etc. After my morning sickness subsided in the second trimester, I went back to the fruits and vegetables. I gained 37 pounds during my pregnancy (and lost 20 immediately after delivery).

I finally hit 37 weeks. I was now out of the woods since 37 weeks is considered full term. We decided to induce at 39 weeks. There is a reason induction may be recommended over the age of 40. Apparently, older women may have lower quality placentas since their eggs are older. Also, placentas start to deteriorate after the pregnancy is full term. So, older women have a double whammy. As the placenta gets near or past the due date, and it starts to deteriorate, this can compromise blood flow to the baby. If the placenta is lower quality to begin with, you could deprive your baby of oxygen which could lead to things like cerebral palsy. Our doctor explained to us that conditions like cerebral palsy usually occur because of a lack of oxygen *during* the pregnancy. Older women may be told induction is recommended because of this risk. Most people have the misconception that this condition usually occurs as a result of a difficult delivery (although that may be true in some cases). Just to be on the safe side, my regular OB sent me back to the perinatologist for a delivery consult. He said the baby looked great, the placenta and amniotic fluid looked great, but he still recommended induction at 39 weeks. He also warned me older women who have never had children have a harder time with cervix dilation and we could try induction, but if I didn't dilate right away, he would recommend a C-Section. I was willing to do whatever was safest for the baby.

My last OB appointment was at 38 weeks, my cervix was already a little dilated which was normal. My OB doctor made arrangements for my induction with the knowledge I might need to go in for a C-section if the natural route didn't work. She was very optimistic I would have a vaginal delivery, especially since I was a little dilated. The next Friday was the big day. I was so scared. I honestly didn't know how on earth I would get a baby out of that narrow opening. I had to keep reminding myself millions of women around the world give birth every day. It *was* possible. Also, the week prior to my induction I could actually feel my pelvic bones moving. This was somewhat painful, but I wanted my body to do what it needed to make room.

The morning of the "big day", we checked into the hospital at 7:00am. I was so anxious I got very little sleep the night before. My husband tried to reassure me that he would be there every step of the way. After all, the baby had to come out one way or the other. After we checked in at the hospital, they started the Pitocin. It actually is quite a slow process. The contractions started quickly, but were so minor for the first 4-5 hours that I really didn't feel anything (it was actually quite boring!) Later, my doctor came in to break my water. I wanted an epidural, but I really hadn't needed it up until that point. Immediately after they broke my water, the contractions intensified. They literally went from a "1" to a "10" on the pain scale in a matter of minutes. I wasn't prepared for that amount of pain and every contraction made me wince and cry. I asked for my epidural but I had to wait since the anesthesiologist was in surgery. Finally, about an hour later, I got my epidural and I immediately felt relief. Although I'm glad I got to experience what labor pains felt like, if I were to do it over again, I would have asked for the epidural *before* they broke my water. I truly admire women who go through natural childbirth. I thought I had a high pain threshold, but labor pains tested my limits!

My cervix totally dilated a few hours later and I began to push. I was progressing, but very slowly. We alternated pushing with "passive descent." This is when you just let the contractions do the work and let the baby come down on its own. Finally about 12 hours after we started the Pitocin, the nurse called the doctor and we were ready to deliver. I wasn't really that tired, even though I'd been pushing for about 4 hours. The doctor looked at me and said "look at me and get mad!" I did and pushed with all my might. We did this for about 30 minutes. Then, finally, with one last push my baby came out. She immediately opened her eyes and stretched her arms out—she was perfect and beautiful! My first thought was that she looked like my husband! I heard a little gurgly cry. Her breathing was slightly labored, so they blew a little oxygen in her face and cleaned out all of her airways and she was fine. Her Apgar scores were great! I had a small first degree laceration which the doctor stitched up after he delivered the placenta and in the meantime my husband went over to the baby and let her squeeze his hand. He commented on how strong her grip was. I got to hold her and get acquainted with her, then she took a short trip to the nursery to make sure her breathing had returned to normal (which it had). They brought her back and I was able to breastfeed her for the first time. Ouch! She really latched on hard! She must have really been hungry.

I later transferred to the mother/baby unit and had an uneventful hospital stay. I must admit, the breastfeeding was harder and more painful than I expected. They should have told me to wear a bra right away since it would have helped with the irritation. I didn't get much sleep in the hospital. All I wanted to do was hold and feed my baby. Additionally, the mother/baby unit is a very noisy place! Even though I had my own room, I could hear all the other babies throughout the night (and I'm sure everyone else could hear mine!)

When I returned home, my husband let me sleep, sleep, sleep. I hadn't had a good night's sleep since before my baby was born and I was really tired after having labored and delivered. I felt much more rested the next day, but I was very swollen and sore. I sat on a doughnut for a couple of weeks and I finally felt well healed enough to start resuming regular activities.

My daughter was (and still is) such a joy. She was a very easy newborn. She ate well, slept well, and had a very calm disposition. I guess us old folks get the easy ones. I never got tired of looking at her or taking care of her. My husband and I took turns with the night feedings and this helped me to get a good night's sleep at least some of the time. People always told me the first month you're on a post-partum "high" and you don't mind the sleep deprivation, but after that, watch out! For me, however, I never came off of the excitement and total absorption of taking care of my baby. Even when I don't get sleep, somehow I just don't seem to mind. In the past, before I had her, any loss of sleep seemed to be a major catastrophe, but not now. To this day, I still look at her and marvel in the miracle – I'm still on the post-partum high! I finally succeeded. I guess deep down, I always knew I would.

Chapter 18
The Joy of Being an Older Parent

I hesitate to talk too much about a successful pregnancy because I know those who are struggling with infertility can feel a sense of being left behind when others get pregnant. However, for me, seeing a "tough case" come to fruition was actually encouraging. Prior to my successful pregnancy, it would hurt my feelings when I heard people talk about how wonderful the experience is. I do understand why they went on and on, but I also try to be sensitive to those that are trying and don't know what's around the next corner.

One good thing about having a less than perfect childhood yourself is you know all of the things you *shouldn't* do. Even at my age, I remember the sinking feeling I had every day when my mother left me in daycare. I know daycare may be a necessity for some people, but if at all possible, try to find a way to stay home with your child/children. There are many books out there on how to make it on one income and how daycare may actually cost you more than staying home. One nice aspect of being an older parent is you may have the financial means to stay home with your baby.

I keep saying us old folks get the easy babies because among other things, my daughter started sleeping through the night at 6 weeks and is still an excellent sleeper. I was envisioning a huge transition when she was born, but somehow, I just worked it in to my day to day life. Yes, life is different, but that's a good thing! I waited 6 long years and I've been rewarded tenfold. I can't begin to tell you the love you feel for this sweet little baby. I honestly think those of us who have struggled with infertility and miscarriage really *do* appreciate more what a miracle the whole process of pregnancy and childbirth is.

I'd be lying if I didn't say I was somewhat of a neurotic mother for the first year of my daughter's life. After dealing with so many miscarriages, it was hard for me to believe I deserved to have everything go so right for once. I had my daughter sleep next to our bed in a bassinet for many months before we made the transition to a crib. Initially, I would constantly check her throughout the night just to make sure I could still hear her breathing. Everything was always fine. The nice thing about having her in the bassinet was she could not roll on her stomach. Babies should sleep on their back for the first year of life to reduce the risk of SIDS. This is more difficult once they move to the crib because there's more room to roll around. You just keep moving them back and hope they'll maintain that position for a while. I think back to the days when my sister's children were babies. The train of thought at that time was you should put babies on their stomach to sleep, and even then, the risk of SIDS was quite small. When babies sleep on their back, the risk is reduced even further.

The hardest part of the first three months was breastfeeding. I wanted to give my baby the best of everything but my nipples actually had broken skin and scabs from small areas of bleeding. I had to begin pumping so my breasts could heal. After about two weeks of pumping I tried to feed her directly from my breast, but she had gotten so comfortable with the bottle, I couldn't get her to switch back. I pumped for three months and after that my milk dried up over a period of 3 to 4 days. I kept trying to pump, but very little would come out. I got my period that same week, so I figured my hormones must have "crashed". I was sorry I could no longer give my baby breast milk, but at least she got it for 3 months. I did not miss the pumping at all.

It is truly one of the most rewarding experiences watching your baby grow and watching her reach each developmental milestone. Everything from smiling to rolling, to sitting, to standing, to walking is just the thrill of a lifetime. In the past, I would see babies do these things all the time, but I never realized just how important and how miraculous it was when you've followed a baby from conception to birth and beyond. It's almost mind boggling how strong the life force is within all of us.

I was a panel member for a group of couples who were going through infertility and/or fertility treatments. Those of us on the panel spoke about our journey through the whole infertility maze. I spoke about everything from IVF, to miscarriage, to deciding on childfree only to get pregnant naturally and carry to term. One thing I was sure to tell the group is you *can* do this. There are so many doctors out there who are negative about older women getting pregnant. I guess they are trying to be honest (from their perspective), but I think the constant negativity older women face about getting pregnant contributes to their inability to get pregnant! *Anything is possible – you just need to tap into the possibilities!*

I know everyone's situation is different, but I've seen some very tough cases succeed. I've also seen many women going through fertility treatment end up getting pregnant naturally during a break. I know a couple of women who were told their FSH was too high and their egg quality was too low and they should look for an egg donor if they wanted to succeed. Two of these women got pregnant naturally -- one while looking for an egg donor, the other while trying to save up enough money to pay for the procedure. One of these women went on to have a second child naturally.

In retrospect, I wouldn't change a thing about my journey to parenthood. With the benefit of hindsight, I can see everything I went through had a purpose and the end result is much better and brighter than I could have ever imagined. If I had been able to get pregnant on the first try, just think what I would have missed out on! I cleaned up my body, my mind, my environment and my life. Not only am I reaping the rewards, so is my husband and my daughter. I truly believe I was not a "victim" of infertility. When you see yourself as a victim, you automatically think there isn't anything you can do to change your situation. Where I am today is the cumulative effect of my past choices. It was my *choice* to delay childbearing, it was my *choice* to throw myself into my career, and it was my *choice* to lead a stressful lifestyle. All of these things ultimately affected my ability to get pregnant. On the other hand, it was my choice to assume responsibility for my fertility. I finally realized that *I* was in control of my body, *not the doctors!* My natural journey to pregnancy has proved to me, once again, that with the right knowledge and commitment, you can achieve anything in life.

Afterword

Since the original publication of this book we have been having a wonderful life with our daughter. Even though we have been asked many times if we are having another child (which is funny given our ages) we always say we are perfectly happy with one. We completely left the "trying to conceive" part of our life behind. I suppose you could say we were "passively" avoiding pregnancy.

You can imagine how surprised I was when, at the age of 49, I found I was pregnant again completely by accident. What's even more amazing was our intercourse was infrequent prior to my conception due to a flu bug which had made its way around our house. Unfortunately, I was miscarrying by the time I even realized I was pregnant. I thought the strange bleeding was the beginning of menopause. Since we were not trying to conceive, this miscarriage was sad but not devastating.

After I knew I miscarried, I went into my doctor's office to get a Rhogam shot (since I'm Rh negative). The nurse administering the shot (who was easily young enough to be my daughter and then some) kept asking me if I wanted some birth control (*Imagine that! Me? On birth control?!*) She said a number of times, "If you still have periods, you can still get pregnant." I didn't go into how I wrote a book on the subject and she was "preaching to the choir" as they say. I politely told her we would be more careful next time. But let this be a lesson to you no matter what your age…*IF YOU STILL HAVE PERIODS, YOU CAN STILL GET PREGNANT!*

Printed in Great Britain
by Amazon